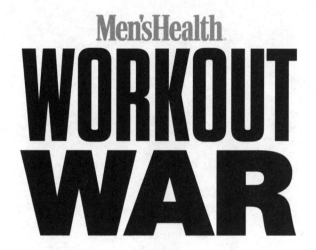

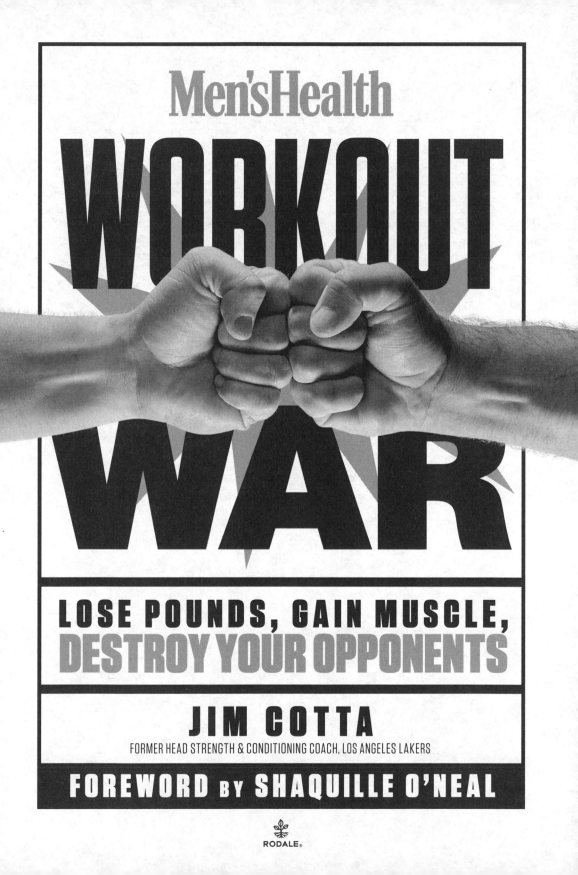

To all of the brave men and women
who serve in the
United States Armed Forces
and to my son Tyler,
*United States Marine.* Get Boozy!

# CONTENTS

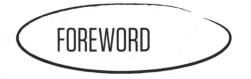
# FOREWORD

**THE BIG SHAMROCK, BIG ARISTOTLE, BIG SHAQTUS, AND THE BIG DIESEL ARE SOME OF MY FAVORITE NICKNAMES FROM MY NBA PLAYING CAREER.** But when Charles Barkley called me the "Big Fat-Ass" while filming TNT's *Inside the NBA*, I got fired up! If he had called me that while on the court, I would have dunked on his ass like 100 times and had him watching the game from the bench. But we're no longer NBA basketball players, so I had to find another way to inflict my Shaq Attack.

At the time, I was in my first year of retirement and about to turn 40. Now don't get me wrong, I'm still dead sexy. But I had put on a few pounds since the years I played for the Los Angeles Lakers and won three Finals MVP Awards. So when Chuck called me out for being fat, I got pissed and said, "Yeah, well you're fat, too, buddy, and I challenge you to a weight-loss competition. Better yet, let's take our shirts off on TV." I thought there was no way Charles would agree to take off his shirt and show off his jelly rolls. But he said, "It's on. Let's do it!" Now I'm not one to ever back down on a challenge, and I have to win. Shoot, I've got four NBA Championship rings; Chuck has *zero*. There was no way I was gonna let this chump beat me.

I knew I needed to call in the strength coach who kept me in shape during my playing days with the Lakers, Jim Cotta. Jim helped me win three straight NBA Championships in 2000, 2001, and 2002 and MVP in the NBA Finals all three of those seasons. Cotta helped keep my body lean and mean during those days in LA, when I averaged 27 points and 12 boards per game, and the years I led the league in field goal percentage for five straight seasons. During those days when training with Jim, I also held the regular season scoring title in 1999 and 2000 and was MVP of the regular season in 2000. I knew I needed to turn back the hands of time to those days when I was in much better shape.

So I got Jim Cotta on board to help me out. Jim is a really smart trainer who knows me all too well. His approach to fitness has always been pretty straightforward: work hard, eat right, and have some fun. Find types of exercise that you enjoy, act like a fool now and then to keep it entertaining, and work out with a purpose or goal. As Jim says, "You need to find your *why*." My *why*? Beat Charles Barkley!

For two months, Jim put me through tough workouts, and I stayed away from fast food and sugar. I dropped 40 pounds; I looked and felt damn good. And the mirror doesn't lie. When I took off my shirt, I was the "Big Sexy" again.

Jim's workout routines and his philosophy of making fitness into a competition is exactly what men need to motivate them to get off the couch and lose some weight. I really enjoyed the daily trash talking with Charles and I know he did, too; it's what kept us motivated.

Hey, every dude on earth wants to look good for the ladies, but most don't have the drive to stick with a fitness plan. This book will give you the tools to get that desire and motivation back while having fun beating up your friends and enemies in a competition.

Can you dig it?!

*Shaquille O'Neal*

# INTRODUCTION

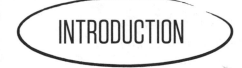

My name is Jim Cotta, and I'm a competition fanatic—a full-blown junkie.

**I'VE BEEN COMPETITIVE EVER SINCE I WAS A CHILD.** I love to watch sports, play sports, bet on sports (and games), and enjoy every facet of a good competition. The game or bet doesn't matter. Whether it's a round of golf with pals, a game of horse, or a quick game of badminton against my kids . . . if there is a winner and a loser, I'm in! Competition gets the juices flowing, no matter the arena. You picked up this book, so my guess is that you're pretty much the same—someone who loves to go head-to-head.

My love of competition is one of the main reasons I decided to become a strength and conditioning coach. After my high school and college football career came to an end, I wanted to help other competitive athletes achieve success on the field and court. Over the years, I've had the pleasure of working with some extremely talented college athletes at the University of Texas and the University of Nevada, Las Vegas. But the highlight of my career came when I joined the Los Angeles Lakers coaching staff in 1997 as the head strength and conditioning coach.

During my time training the Lakers, I got to work with some of the best basketball players in the world. Under the incredible coaching philosophy of Phil Jackson, we made history a second time by winning our second three-peat (back-to-back-to-back) NBA World Championships (2000, 2001, and 2002). It was an amazing time in my life. Being part of the Lakers dynasty was incredible. I was constantly amazed by the wisdom of Coach Jackson. He could motivate guys in ways that no one else could, always keeping in mind that competition brings out the best effort in men. I did my best to follow his example by bringing that same kind of philosophy, work ethic, and respect to my weight room.

I took our games—and my job—personally; I did everything within my power to ensure my guys were in top shape when they hit the court. I shared in the emotions of every team win and loss. We had an 82-game schedule. I spent more time with guys like Shaquille O'Neal, Robert Horry, Rick Fox, and Derek Fisher than I did my own family. The players were like family to me. My life revolved around the team and my guys.

# YOU DON'T KNOW WHAT YOU'VE GOT UNTIL IT'S GONE

When I decided to leave the Lakers in 2004 to spend more time with my own family, I thought I was closing the door on that part of my life. However, after a while, I realized that a small piece of me was missing.

Can you guess what it was?

Yeah, competition. I missed the motivation of competition and the fear of losing. When my wife, Amy, said she thought I should work with golfers, helping them to compete on a higher level, I was intrigued and excited. I soon started taking on clients and quickly built a reputation for being the go-to guy in Nashville for golf fitness.

Most of my clients are Average Joe golfers who go out there every week, competing and gambling against their buddies. But like my pro athletes, they are willing to do whatever it takes to get the job done and win every round. That rekindled the passion I left in LA.

Then in 2012, Shaq called me up and asked if I would help him win a bet he made with Charles Barkley. These basketball giants were going to compete to see who could lose the most weight, and then take their shirts off on national television. It was such a crazy idea that I jumped on the chance. And it was a blast! For 2 months, I lived and traveled with Shaq, working every minute of every day with one sole purpose—to help him crush Charles Barkley on national TV.

Every Thursday night while taping the NBA on TNT, I would sit in the studio watching and listening to those two knuckleheads go at it (on and off camera), taunting one another about their weight and who was going to win the competition; that's when the lightbulb went off in my head. I suddenly knew the secret to sticking with a fitness program! I had found the solution to America's weight problem. It's been right here in front of our faces this whole time, and none of us ever realized it!

# BUILD IT AND THEY WILL COME

You have to be somewhat of a book and research nerd to be successful in my business. But as much as I love science, I know it doesn't motivate people. Over the years, I have seen an array of new diets, exercise fads and trends, changes in research, and new research results. Over the last several years in particular, there's been an explosion of new fitness equipment, diets, supplements, online training devices and resources, different types and styles of one-on-one personal training, and group fitness classes. At no other time in history have we had so many health and fitness tools at our fingertips. We've never known more about food; how the body processes it; or which foods to eat to lower our body fat, lose weight, and increase our overall health. The amount of nutrition information in the media is mind-boggling!

Have you ever noticed how many liposuction and weight-loss clinics there are? Not to mention the increase in doctors' offices offering hormone replacement as a way to lose weight and regain youthful vigor. It seems like everyone is searching for the *magic pill*, and businesses are offering quick-fix solutions like never before.

Yet with all of that at our disposal, our nation is getting fatter and fatter. Guys, it's not just the women packing on the pounds; we are, too. It's estimated that 83 percent of men in the United States will be overweight or obese by 2020. That's right—83 percent! And that's both scary and sad.

So what's the problem? Why are people motivated to lose hundreds of pounds on television shows, but they won't do it on their own? How is it that we know what to do, but we won't do it? We've been missing the *stimulation factor*, that's what! Unless there is money or a huge reward on the line, the motivation isn't there.

## STIMULATION ISN'T JUST FOR THE BEDROOM

I think most of us could agree that society and social media have conditioned us to crave constant stimulation and instant gratification. If something isn't fun or immediate, we tend to lose focus and interest. If we find exercise, an eating plan, or anything else in our lives boring, we say, "What's the point?" and we quit.

### WHAT'S BETTER THAN SEX FOR MOTIVATION?

Okay, maybe not better ... but damn close?

Competition!

Come on, admit it: You're not thinking about sex during the Super Bowl. Heck, during the last few minutes of a nail-biter of a basketball game, you'd probably choose watching three-pointers over the prospect of a threesome. Well, maybe not, but you get the point: We men love a good dose of competition, and it doesn't matter if we're in it or viewing it from the stands or watching it on TV; we've got to have it.

## LIFE IS LIKE *SEINFELD*

A great example of our competitive nature can be seen in the iconic episode of *Seinfeld* called "The Competition." Here's how the storyline goes: George's mother catches him in a very compromising, personal situation, after which George, Jerry, Kramer, and Elaine stage a contest to see who can go the longest without sexual gratification.

"You'll be out before we get the check!" Jerry taunts Kramer.

As with anything else in life, one by one, they all face obstacles that try to throw them off track. Jerry sees a woman in the apartment across the street constantly walking around naked. Plus, Jerry's virgin girlfriend is ready to have sex. George visits his injured mother in the hospital, where a sexy-sounding female patient with a tantalizing profile enjoys a sponge bath by a female nurse on the other side of the curtain. And Elaine finds out that John F. Kennedy Jr. has a crush on her. One by one, they all start falling out of the competition.

This episode of *Seinfeld* pokes fun at how men (and Elaine, in this case) will challenge each other and bet on anything and everything, including sex! We'll fight off any amount of temptation, because we must win. And we definitely can't allow ourselves to be the first loser or the last-place finisher.

This is the very reason I built a competition around the fitness and nutrition component of this book. I knew if I wrote a book that was a stand-alone 60-day program, you might read it or you might not. You might use it for a week or two, then lose your motivation and throw in the towel, because you don't have a powerful enough reason to chase your goal. I knew if you could make a small wager on your effort, compete against your buddies, smack talk about it, and share a few laughs during the process, you'd do it—and you'd stick to it.

## GET REAL

Let's not kid ourselves here, fellas—we're men, and men don't diet. We're never going to follow some flowery, pink program designed by and for women. It just isn't going to happen. And we're sure as hell not going to invite one another to join in on the latest group fitness class craze, like Zumba or a Weight Watchers meeting (not that there's anything wrong with that). The fitness-diet industry just hasn't figured out yet how guys tick, though. That's why we don't participate in their estrogen-based nonsense. Instead, we're going to do things *our way*.

Let's get to work.

Put down that remote, Wilma, and grab a pair of dumbbells!

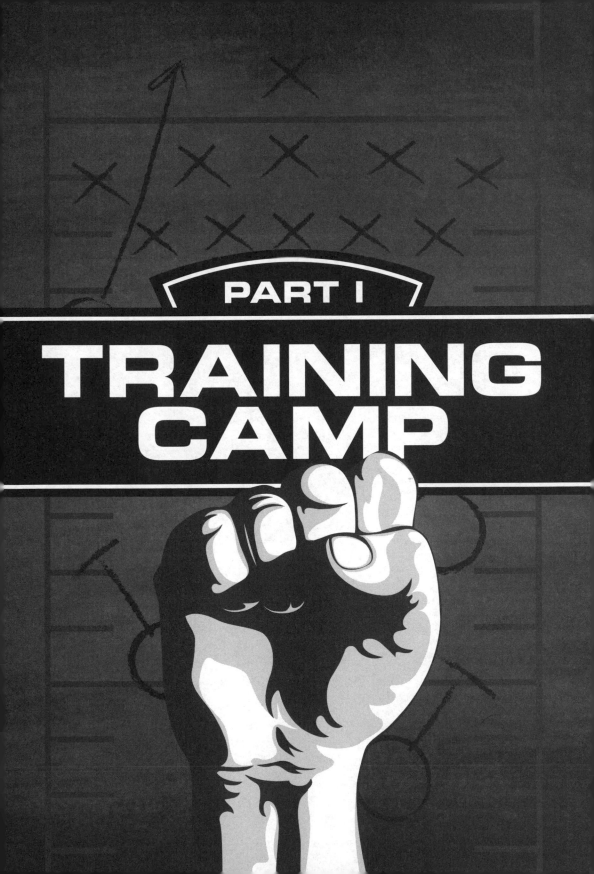

# PART I
# TRAINING CAMP

# WARMUPS

## HOW TO START A WORKOUT WAR

**WELCOME TO THE SEVENTH LEVEL OF HELL, LADIES . . .** Buckle up your chinstraps, 'cause it's about to get real. Forget everything you *think* you know about diet and fitness programs.

You're about to enter the *NO* Zone:

**No** gimmicks

**No** BS

**No** fancy health clubs

**No** marathon, 90-minute workouts

We're changing the game.

We are going to train hard. Sweat like pigs. Compete like gladiators and kick major amounts of ass.

I'm joking, *sort of.* Hopefully you'll find this book easy to use and easy to read. I tried to keep everything simple and straight to the point. You'll find some sections that require a little reading, while others you can quickly scan to get the needed information. And for those who don't like to read, I put the information into visual graphics and cheat sheets for you. So you have no excuses for not succeeding.

I wrote this book with one thing in mind—*competition*! I purposely kept the in-depth science on the light side so you have more time to do the competition instead of reading about *why* something is the way that it is. This means you're *not* going to find mounds of text and research on things like how much protein to eat, the different chambers of the heart, or the difference between the fast-twitch and slow-twitch muscle fibers. I figured if you really want to know the scientific facts on a particular subject, you'll Google it.

# WHO THIS BOOK IS FOR

This book is for the millions of American men who are tired of being out of shape or overweight. It's for those who want to get back to playing the sports they love instead of just spectating, for guys who miss the adrenaline rush of competition and the camaraderie that accompanies a competitive athletic pursuit.

Most of us know the path to a healthier life: Eat better and exercise more. The tough part is finding the motivation to do it. That's the problem this book fixes. By awakening our innate competitive nature, the will to win (or at least not lose) serves as the ultimate motivating factor, 'cause let's face it—as a man, you *must* win; it's all about winning and bragging rights.

An increasing number of people are turning to placing formal wagers with friends or coworkers to reach their weight-loss goals. A study in a recent issue of the *Journal of the American Medical Association* found that people who had financial incentives to lose weight were much more successful at dieting than those who did not.

Games, sports, you name it; even if there isn't cash involved, competition drives interest and action, too. Imagine if we put the

# COMPETITION =
## MOTIVATION

same effort into eating right and exercising as we do fantasy football or March Madness (the research, the stats, the changing lineup, not to mention the countless hours of watching games that we have no interest in, other than the fact that there are financial implications based on the outcome). If we put that kind of passion into eating healthy and exercising, we'd look as ripped as Terrell Owens.

Competition is deeply rooted in our male DNA. It helped us survive when we were carrying clubs instead of laptops, and it's how we measure ourselves against other men today. Whether we're the ones playing the game or just betting on the game, our lust for competition makes us do crazy things. It doesn't matter if it's ping-pong, horseshoes, rec softball, or working out—we will do anything and everything in our power to make sure that we come out on top.

Not convinced? Just think of all the dumb bets you've placed in your lifetime. I once bet a friend $100 that he couldn't run to the top of a sand hill without stopping, and he didn't hesitate to give it a shot. I won the bet!

Winning to us is often more important than the challenge itself. Our self-esteem hinges upon it. Sometimes this means beating others, and sometimes this simply means beating our own previous best effort. Anyone who has ever run that lonely oval of a high school track with an eye on his beat-up stopwatch or shiny new iPhone gets what it means to compete against himself. (How many times have you heard a friend or coworker brag about how fast he could run a mile in high school, and you know that now he couldn't crack 12 minutes if his life depended on it?) And maybe, just maybe, the single most important reason we want to win is for the bragging rights. But money is great, too.

# SHOW ME THE MONEY! $ $$

Even pro athletes are motivated to work out because of money. Many professional sports teams fine players for missing a workout or give guys bonuses during the off-season if they show up for all the workouts. It's hard to believe that a player making $10 million a year would be upset over a fine for a missed workout, but they are, and it gets them to show up for the training sessions. If you threaten to take money out of their pockets, it wakes them up and motivates them.

You would think an athlete who is playing a sport at the highest level, in front of millions of fans, would be motivated enough to train like a beast all the time, but that's not always the case.

If you and your buddies are getting bored with the same-old, tired daily routine, this could be your new thing. Your wife or significant other might complain about your spending too much time and energy on fantasy football, golf, or poker, but you won't find them complaining about your spending time getting in shape and wrapping it all up with a fun reunion or party somewhere to celebrate the hard work you put in. Consider it your new "bro" time. Maybe it can replace your slow-pitch, beer-drinking, after-work softball league for just one season while you get your "house" in order.

You might consider using a get-back-in-shape competition as an opportunity to get your high school football teammates or college fraternity brothers back together. You can take your contest online and participate with your buddies from all over the country or the world. You're going to be taking a large portion of this mission online anyway, so whether most of your competitors or teammates are local or spread out, Facebook and other social networking media are going to play a large part.

If most of your teammates or competitors live in different regions, the winning team should have some added incentive to win, besides the greenbacks. Maybe it's time for you and your crew—as scattered as you are—to have a reunion. Win or lose, you and your closest buds can agree to meet in person to celebrate when all is said and done.

Your workplace offers another great opportunity as a contest hub. If you own the company, would you like to cut the cost of your employees' health care while possibly increasing productivity?

Starting a Workout War competition at your company is the perfect way to create a fun workplace, boost morale, improve the health of employees, and even increase performance.

According to a Gallup Poll conducted in 2011, full-time employees who are overweight, obese, or who have chronic health issues miss around *450 million days per year* over that of their healthy coworkers. This equates to about $153 billion in lost productivity every year. A recent study by the American College of Cardiology showed that those who either were paid every month for losing weight or had to pay if they didn't lose weight were more likely to reach their weight-loss goals. Talk to your human resources department about your interest in starting a Men's Health Workout War fitness and weight-loss competition; it could earn you major brownie points with your boss.

# HOW TO USE THE BOOK

If you have the time, I suggest thumbing through the pages to familiarize yourself with the book. Feel free to read over anything that catches your eye as you scan. You can read through the book before implementing the competition or you can dive right in and follow the step-by-step instructions for building a competition in real time as you read. Here's a list of what you'll be doing to get this thing going:

## COMPETITION CHEAT SHEET

**Step 1.** Scouting: Think about who you want to compete against—friends, coworkers, and family.

**Step 2.** Choose a type of competition: What will you be measuring?

**Step 3.** Select a competition format—head-to-head, teams, or eliminations. Decide on a buy-in amount (and/or tentative prizes for winner and/or loser). Choose your tracking system.

**Step 4.** Set a start and end date.

**Step 5.** Recruit competitors.

**Step 6.** Set parameters and rules.

**Step 7.** Crank it up! Send out reminders, collect fees, and assign refs or a banker.

**Step 8.** Host a kickoff event for weigh-in, before photos, or other measurements.

Once you set up your Workout War, it's time to get down to individual preparation. When it comes time to do the actual 60-day workout and eating plan, which are detailed in Part II, keep in mind that you'll be training and eating in the quarter that you're currently living in. So stay in the moment and don't get too far ahead of yourself. You can look ahead to the next quarter, but don't jump ahead. The training principles behind the workouts get progressively harder as the quarters go by, and you need to work your way up to them, or else you're gonna be hurting.

## KEEP IT OR KICK IT

As you'll see in Chapter 3, you'll be given many ideas on how to run your competition. Feel free to keep and use any of the information that I've laid out for you. Follow what you like verbatim; use what you want and kick the rest to the street. I'm here to help you start and run a competition, not split hairs on the perfect way to run your contest. It's your game, boss. Drive it!

## BAIT THE TRAP

As you're reading Chapter 2 and getting to know the book, this is a great time to start baiting the traps by putting out little teaser e-mails, Facebook page posts, and tweets to get people wondering what you're up to. Send your recruits to MensHealth.com/WorkoutWar for exercise tips and competition advice.

Make sure to use some hashtags (#) and FB tag @MensHealth @MHWW so we can repost and retweet you. Yes, now you can also use hashtags on Facebook. Tag your friends and tag me. My personal Twitter account is @CottaBelieve.

You could tweet and post things like:

> "I'm about to unleash world domination @YourFriendsTwitter."
>
> "Who wants in? #MensHealth #WeightWorkoutWar @CottaBelieve."
>
> "I'm going to be a Lean, Mean, Fighting Machine in 60 Days! @MensHealthmag."
>
> "Who wants a 6-pack? Of ABS! Game on! #MHWW."
>
> "I'm about to become the next Lou Ferrigno. @WeightWorkoutWar."
>
> "I will be taking your money and looking like Arnold. #MHWW."

You'll want to keep up with the social media taunting after your competition starts. You can send out funny pictures of fat guys and say they are one of your competition buddies. You can tweet and post motivational photos and quotes. And, of course, you'll want to brag often about your Rival Strength Challenge scores (you'll learn about these later) and how you're crushing everyone else! For example:

> "Do you hear that? That's me crushing @YourFriendsTwitter #MHRivalChallenge #B52 time!"
>
> "BAM that just happened! 20 rounds of #99Problems. Suck it @YourFriendsTwitter #MHRivalChallenge."

For more help with social media, see the Workout War Social Media Cheat Sheet on page 20.

# WHAT'S WHAT

Here's the rundown of what you'll find in the pages that follow:

## PART I—TRAINING CAMP

**Chapter 1: Warmups.** You're already there.

**Chapter 2: Scouting Report.** This chapter suggests ways to find players to fill out your competition.

**Chapter 3: Game Plan: Build Your Contest** provides step-by-step instructions for setting up your own Workout War, from choosing a competition format and establishing rules and dates to organizing a kickoff.

## PART II—PLAYBOOK

**Chapter 4: Sweat to Win: The Muscle-Up Plan** explains the breakdown of the four-quarter (plus overtime), 60-day workout plan.

**Chapter 5: The Exercises.** Here you'll find all the exercises with instructional photographs used in Part III Game Day.

**Chapter 6: The Lean-Out Meal Plan** delivers the skinny on the diet and nutrition program you can use to devour your competition.

**Chapter 7: The Lean-Out Recipes.** This is your go-to spot for fuel—tasty meals that supply energy and muscle-building protein and kick junk calories to the curb.

## PART III—GAME DAY

This section's five chapters, broken down by four quarters and an overtime period, outline the daily workouts for each of the 12 days in the quarter and include suggested meal plans and helpful shopping lists for that particular quarter.

## UNLEASH YOUR INNER RAMBO

No matter what brought you here—whether it's better health, pride, taunting, or a good dose of competition—you've come to the right place. This program has the potential to change your life! Grab the opportunity now. Before you skip to the exercises and meal plans, read over Chapter 3 to start thinking about the type of competition you want to run and how to get started. Then jump in with both feet.

# SCOUTING REPORT ②

## FIND AND RECRUIT THE PLAYERS

**THIS CHAPTER IS YOUR TOOLBOX FOR BUILDING *YOUR* COMPETI-
TION.** I emphasize *YOUR* because it's your game. I'm merely here to
motivate and guide. Don't feel as if you have to use all the tools here.
Make the game as simple or as complex as you like. If you come up
with an idea that's not listed, and it rings your bell, run with it. There
is more than one way to skin a cat, or in this case, shed some *fat*. The
idea here is to take what excites you and blow it up and make it fun.

If you're the first of your friends to read this book, then it's on
your shoulders to get the ball rolling. Like a good sports scout, it's
your job to go out into the world and draft cronies to take on the
challenge with you—as the leader and commander. But first, you

# DRAFT YOUR FRIENDS AND LEAD THE CHARGE INTO A FRIENDLY FITNESS COMPETITION. UNLEASH YOUR INNER RAMBO. KICK ASS. LEAVE NO SURVIVORS.

have to rally *your* own inner troops. You've got to want this. You've got to be the General Patton of this competition. You've got to exude enthusiasm and leadership. Only then will others really be ready to take your lead. Got it?

You can draft (sucker, shame, or bribe) people from anywhere and everywhere to join the challenge. Depending on how large you want to grow your competition, everyone within the group can also become a scout, recruiting his friends to join in before the start date. You'll start by rallying your compadres with an e-mail invitation/challenge like the sample shown opposite. Send them to MensHealth.com/WorkoutWar for more information. Here's how it'll go down (again, adjust as you see fit). Let the fun begin!

Let's take a closer look at steps involving scouting, recruiting, drafting, and lighting the competitive fire under your players.

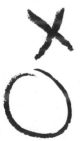

## SCOUTING

Time to recruit your victims, I mean . . . competitors.

This just might be the easiest part of the process. Think about all the people you know, and all the people they know. Trust me, when I ran a test group for this book, within a week I had all kinds of people

# DEAR FRIENDS,

**I CHALLENGE** you to a contest (against me and others) to lose weight (or get ripped) and get healthy. The competition will run for 60 days and is based on the percentage of weight lost. Each competitor will pay [insert amount] to enter the contest. Whoever loses the most weight wins the pot! This could mean some major cash for one of us.

I'm sure we could all use a kick in the pants to get motivated to work out more and eat healthier. We will be following the Workout War exercise and nutrition plan in the book *Men's Health Workout War*. It will provide us the tools needed to look better, feel better, manage stress, sleep better, and lose weight. The contest will be calculated in a way that is fair to everyone—even those who don't have a lot of excess weight to lose.

I have tentatively set the start date for [enter date]. If you want to look and feel better while winning some cold, hard cash, then join in. Once we get closer to the start date, I will send you a follow-up e-mail with more details.

## I look forward to
# KICKING YOUR ASS!

[Your name]

wanting in on the action—women included—but I told the ladies no! You will get this, too, but tell the women they can't join. No wives. No girlfriends. No compromises. No surrender. This is something for the guys. Women have their groups and do boot camp, Zumba, yoga, and Pilates and yap at the coffee shop afterward. This one is strictly for *men*!

You can find competitors anywhere, but in case you're having trouble, I made a list of types of people to look for and places to find them. Now here's the thing—if you plan on doing a money pool for the winner, the more people you have to participate, the larger the winner's pot. So keep that in mind when you're out recruiting participants and let them know what the pot could possibly be. You tell any guy that a pot is over $1,000, they'll be like, "Where do I sign up!?"

Don't ever be shy about telling people what you are doing (or about the money!). You'll be surprised; the sheer mention of this competition will make guys want to jump in headfirst.

# WHO TO SCOUT: EVERYONE'S YOUR COMPETITION

To help get the competitive juices flowing, I've put together a list of the different types of guys that would be game to *get into the game*. I'm willing to wager that as you read through this list, you can think of at least two guys who fall within each of these categories.

**Mr. Social:** This is the guy who knows everyone—he's never met a stranger. His list of contacts is a mile long, and he's not afraid to reach out to them. This is your go-to guy to help you scout!

**The athlete:** This guy currently participates in athletics or longs to be back in the shape of his glory years. He still talks about that one spectacular play he made at his high school football game. Or he actually was a college athlete at one point, but has definitely let himself go a bit. He will want in . . . guaranteed!

**The meathead:** These evolutionary-hindered, sleeveless wonders are down with anything and everything that they believe will increase the girth of their biceps and pecs.

**The rookie:** Those who are new to the fitness game are intimidated by the weight room and are not sure how to work out properly. However, they are in the market for a fun new way to get into shape and drop a few pounds.

**The geezer:** The middle-aged guys—don't count them out! A recent study by psychologists from the University of Oregon showed that nearly 70 percent of men aged 45 to 54 chose to go head-to-head with an opponent. This group of men is more competitive than any of the other groups. If they're unmarried, they're still trying to look good for women, believing that they can still land a twenty-something hottie. Those who are married will be looking to spice up the bedroom action.

**The smack talker:** They are always looking for new ways to light their buddies up and let them have it. They love to talk shit! These guys thrive on the thrill of competition. There are basically two things these guys like to brag about . . . and competition is the other one.

**The bookie:** These guys run the office pool. They're not shady, but they sure do love the smell of greenbacks and good competition. Let's face it, guys will bet on anything—like in the movie *Caddyshack*, where the guys were betting on whether Spaulding would pick his nose, then betting again on whether or not he would eat it. Bookies are great at rallying the troops for some good, old-fashioned competitive fun and gambling.

**The statistician:** Most guys will fall under this category. They love numbers and measuring their improvements. These guys are the reason fantasy football exists!

**The wannabe:** The funniest of all the groups. These guys may not even enjoy or think about working out, but they want to hang with the cool kids. Since the whole office is doing it, they'll follow the other sheep and jump into the challenge with both feet.

*C'mon dude!*

**The skeptic:** This naysayer doesn't believe anything will ever get him back in shape, and that's been his excuse for years. But like the wannabe, he's willing to go along for the ride. He's not about to turn down a good bet or challenge to show off his peacock feathers.

**The country clubber:** Don't think they're timid just because they wear plaid shorts and lug golf clubs. Golfers love, love, love to gamble! These guys are beasts in sheep's clothing. Like the bookies, geezers, and wannabes, this group of guys is down for anything that pits them head-to-head with one another. They may also be secretly seeking out a way to reignite their home life, hoping that getting in shape will help. Gee, you think?

**The freak:** You know these guys. They are the crazy-eyed nut bags who you'll find on any given weekend running through mud and fire wearing a kilt to be crowned the next warrior. These guys actively search the Internet for Spartan-type races to prove their prowess.

See? Just about everyone is a potential depositor of their hard-earned money into your personal bank account. Now let's look at where to find these guys and how to get them to take the bait.

**Close friends:** Don't worry about the list getting too big, because not everyone is going to want in. If you really want it to grow, then encourage all your friends to send invites (or forward e-mails) to anyone they think would want to get in. Don't overthink this by saying to yourself, "Well, Dave doesn't have that much weight to lose," or "Greg hates to work out." Who cares? This is a competition with a prize—it's gambling! Whatever you want to call it, people will want in. Trust me.

**Family members:** If you have family members who are cool enough to take the heat, then by all means ask them to join. Now, on the other hand, if you plan on getting down and dirty and don't want your family to know how you truly roll with your buddies, you might want to keep them out this round.

**Coworkers/workplace:** If your workplace is where you think most of the people are going to come from, then maybe the first place to start is your boss's office and let him know you're thinking about starting this competition. Tip: Have the competition specifics organized before this meeting. You want to look buttoned up just as you would going into an important meeting. Besides, if you sell this to your boss correctly, he or she may throw some more money into the winner's pot. Tell your boss how this is a great way for people to get healthier, promotes good team building (which is code for trash talking), adds to productivity at work (instead of ducking out early to hit happy hour, then coming to work the next day with a hangover), encourages fewer sick days, and gives employees more energy.

The whole corporate wellness thing has been big for a while, because everyone knows the benefits of having healthy employees. But even when they build you a nice fancy gym at work, hire trainers to show you what to do, and give you an incentive like saving $50 on your insurance if you show up at the gym twice a week, employees still lose their motivation. But if the boss puts up a thousand bucks, added to the $50 everyone else had to pay to get in on the competition, and the winner takes all (or even if the top three get money), that'll provide some serious motivation for people to eat healthy and work out hard.

**High school or college buds:** Depending on how long you've been out of school, none of you are probably the hunks you once thought you were. It's not likely that time has been nice to your hairline or your waistline.

This is a great group of guys to kindle the spirit of competition with. Chances are you all have a lot of skeletons in your closets that would make for great smack-talking material. Not to mention, if you have an upcoming reunion or golf outing, a dose of 60-day competition might be just what you need leading up to your reunion. The final weigh-in could be during your get-together.

**Church or other social clubs:** Gatherings are great places to find people. Now you may be thinking to yourself, *No, that's not right, I shouldn't ask anyone that I know through the church.* Trust me, the

Lord wants us to be healthy and show a little more respect for our bodies. Look at it this way—you are helping someone who is over-weight; by getting them in on the competition, you may be adding years to their life. If God could add another Commandment to the Ten, it might be, "Thou shalt not be a lard ass."

**Neighborhood or apartment complex:** Even if you don't know your neighbors very well, throw up a sign and see if anyone responds. Give it a shot and maybe you'll meet some cool guys who love a good competition.

**Facebook friends:** Facebook is an awesome place to dig up old buddies and have your friends easily recruit for you, via their tribe (FB friends). You want to talk about leverage? With Facebook, you can reach people from all over your city or the country that you don't even know, if you want to go that route. You can also turn your wife or girlfriend into a scout for you. Have her post something on her Facebook page about the competition you're starting and leverage her friends' husbands, boyfriends, and family members.

**Twitter and blog followers:** In the event that you're a blogger of sorts, your tribe (followers) is a great place to go mining. Now if you're a financial expert, for example, you want to be careful about not turning off your followers or potential customers. So if you want it to be a full-out trash-talking war, you should keep it to people you know personally. On the other hand, if you want to keep the competition in calmer waters and use this as a way to build loyalty among your tribe, this would be a great way to do it.

**Fantasy pool members:** Do I really need to say anything here? These guys have money burning a hole in their pockets. Put the bet out there and they'll bite. If you are in any kind of sports pool—football, basketball, golf, whatever—reach out to those guys. You already know that they love to be in a pool.

**Health and sports club:** Unless you live on Muscle Beach in California, it's not likely that everyone with a gym or health club membership in your area is already a chiseled Adonis. Not only are you going to find

# 8 Ways to Recruit

Announce in workplace newsletter
Post flyers in workroom
Word of mouth
Phone calls
Facebook
Twitter
E-mail
Text

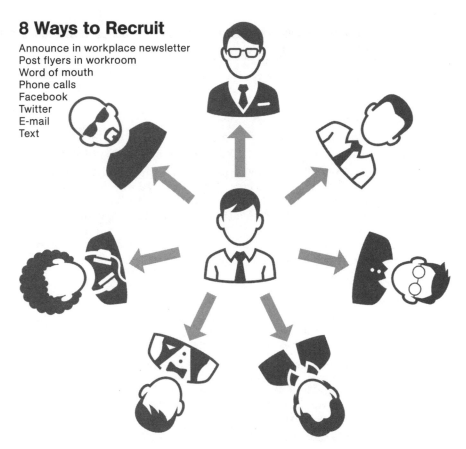

guys who need to shape up, but you'll also be surprised at how many of them would love the motivation of a competition to get into shape.

Make sure to give special attention to any friend or relative who has the potential to be a great recruiter; you can't do this all by yourself, so put others to work. You know the guy—he talks to everyone like a car salesman and knows everyone in town. You've got to get that guy on board. Know someone whose job has contact with a lot of people on a daily basis? What about the friend who is a regular golfer or is a member of a country club? He will also be a great recruiter for you. Like I stated earlier, golfers are competitive and love a good wager. Why do you think they spend so much time on the course? These guys could land you another ten competitors, easily. More competitors equals more money for you when you win!

*(continued on page 22)*

# Workout War Social Media Cheat Sheet

You've got to engage to enrage your competition, and social media is a great way to do that publicly!

## Twitter Basics

1. Open an account at www.twitter.com.
2. Create a Twitter handle. You can use your actual name or anything you like. For example, mine is @CottaBelieve; my wife uses her name @AmyCotta, but then uses @Imove for her business and the hashtag #medalsofhonor to promote her nonprofit.
3. Start following your friends and other people, things, or interests.
4. Recruit followers by letting them know you've become a new resident of Twitterville.
5. Limit tweets to 120 characters: You can do up to 140 characters within a post; however, try to keep it to 120 so people can retweet you.

### THE LINGO

| | |
|---|---|
| @ | Reply: This is the way you talk via Twitter. Without it, whomever you are trying to reach might not see your post. Example: @Strongman Thanks for the great workout today! |
| # | Hashtag: Use this symbol to tag things of importance and to find trending topics. When users search for a topic or click on a #trending topic, they'll be able to see what's going on in the Tweetosphere. Using hashtags is a great way to get more views of your tweet and start conversations. |
| DM | Direct message: This is a way of having a private conversation on Twitter. You must be following someone in order to send a DM. |
| RT | Retweet: RT shows that you are posting something from another user. Retain @Username in front of the retweeted text to show who originally sent it. For example: RT @CottaBelieve It's time to get your fat ass off the couch! @NameofFoeYouWantToTag#MHWW. |
| #FF | Follow Friday: Using hashtags, you can recommend other people to follow your followers. |

## Facebook Basics

1. Join Facebook at www.facebook.com.
2. Set up a personal or professional profile page.
3. Upload any photos or personal information you would like to share and set your security settings to whatever you like. Security settings are where you can limit who can see your posts and photos.
4. Set up a Facebook group (if you want) for your competition. Setting up a "secret group" will allow only invited members to participate and see posts. This gives competitors a safe place to harass each other in private.

5. Like and join pages of interest like *Men's Health* and Workout War for updates, news, and events.

6. Hashtags and handles are now allowed on Facebook, so you can use them like you do with Twitter.

## THE LINGO

| Like | This is a way of letting people know that you appreciate or "like" a particular post or page. |
|------|----------------------------------------------------------------------------------------------|
| Status | This is the empty box where you get to write what's on your mind or to share photos, videos, links, or anything you want your friends to see and comment on. As of the writing of this book, Facebook now allows hashtags. |
| Message | This is a way of sending a private message to either an individual or a group of people. |

## YouTube Basics

1. Set up a YouTube account at www.youtube.com.

2. Create your own Workout War contest channel at www.youtube.com/.

3. Upload your Rival Strength Challenge videos. Remember to tag @MensHealthMag @MHWW

4. Connect with others by viewing, liking, subscribing, and commenting on their videos.

## THE LINGO

| Like | On YouTube, you can rate videos by using the thumbs-up or -down button. |
|------|------------------------------------------------------------------------|
| View | This refers to how many people have viewed a particular video. |
| Subscribe | This shows how many people are following a page or channel. When you subscribe to a page, you'll be updated when new videos are uploaded. |

# MORE TIPS ON RECRUITING COMPETITORS

## PROD THE CATTLE

You've sent out your initial e-mails and communication about the challenge. After a few days, send out a follow-up e-mail, post, or direct text to those who need a little more encouraging to join the competition. Facebook and other social media can make it easier to drum up "cheerleaders" for you or your team along the way. Get family and friends of each competitor online to cajole, cheer, jeer, and encourage you as you post milestones or obstacles. If you had a killer week of success, let them know! In other words, don't just post about this to get the ball rolling; keep the social media thread going, guys.

Now remember, in addition to the e-mails, Facebook posts, and texts, make sure you follow up with the guys who will help the most with the recruiting. Take 'em out for a beer and get 'em fired up about how much fun this is gonna be. Give them a title like "Associate General Manager of the 'No More Fatties' Competition of 2015." Something that makes them feel important. Make phone calls to anyone who responds to an e-mail or Facebook post that says, "I'm in," to get them even more amped and to tell them to get out there and recruit. (Remember your ABCs: A=Always, B=Be, C=Closing. Always Be Closing!) Every guy you come into contact with during the course of the day is a potential competitor. If they show even mild interest, get their e-mail address and send them an invite into the competition.

Before you know it, you will have plenty of people to get this thing going. If you don't want too many people, then set a limit on it—maybe 15 people. This will motivate people to commit also, by saying the first 15 people who commit to this are in—everyone else can hit the bricks.

Now get to work and recruit.

# GAME PLAN

## NAIL THE DETAILS OF YOUR COMPETITION

**YOU'VE STARTED SOME BUZZ AMONG YOUR BUDDIES.** Now get down to creating the structure of your competition. Start by asking yourself some questions. What kind of competition do you want to create? How many competitors are you looking to recruit? What will motivate you to build your best body ever? (After all, you're doing all this for number one, aren't you?)

There are a lot of ways to go with this, and they all can be fun. I personally find the small-group approach to be the most fun, especially when it's done among really good friends. But any size contest can work.

Here are some ways to structure your Workout War.

# CHOOSE A TYPE OF COMPETITION

**Head-to-head:** It's just you and your counterpart. Man versus man, brother versus brother, winner takes the pie. This is the easiest type of contest to organize.

**The small group (2 to 10 individuals):** This is the next easiest to manage because of its size. It's ideal for an intimate competition among friends. With this size, it's typically winner take all.

**The big group (10 or more individuals):** With a larger group, you can get creative with your prizes. Depending on the number of players recruited, you can establish prize money for the top three, five, or ten competitors.

**Teams:** Teams are a great way to even the playing field if some people don't have much weight to lose. In this scenario, you combine individual results into a team score that reflects a percentage of weight lost, total inches lost, or other measurements. Team competition brings another level of motivation to the game since you'll have the support and encouragement of your teammates to keep you going. You can work out and even eat together to keep one another on the up and up. Teams could have captains who pick from the list of competitors, just like when you were a kid playing kickball. And this time, it's the fat "kid" who will probably get picked first.

**Last man standing elimination:** This works best with a large group of competitors. In this format, every 2 weeks you could have a weigh-in measuring either pounds or percentage of weight lost in which one-quarter of the competitors are eliminated from the competition. So let's say you have 20 guys in the competition. At the first weigh-in, the bottom five are booted out. Then 2 weeks later, the next bottom five get cut. At the third weigh-in, five more are out, leaving five guys for the final weigh-in to decide the winner.

**Last team standing elimination:** Team elimination can be run the same as above, and you can adjust the number of weeks based on how many teams you've recruited. Let's say you had four teams. You could do the first weigh-in at the 4-week mark, and the bottom team is out, leaving you with three teams. Do another weigh-in at the 6-week point; bottom team is out, leaving you with two teams. The final two teams have a weigh-in at the end—the 8-week mark—to determine the winner.

**Bracket elimination (individual):** A bracket competition runs just like the March Madness college basketball brackets do. This works best if you have either 4, 8, 16, 32, or 64 competitors. Put the names in a hat and draw to fill out the bracket randomly or rank the individuals as in the college basketball tournament by how much over weight they are. In this competition, you go head-to-head with whoever is in your bracket. At the 2-week weigh-in, whoever wins moves on to the next round's weigh-in 2 weeks later. You go until you are down to two people and can crown a weight-loss champion.

**Bracket elimination team:** Same as above, but with teams.

**Calcutta:** The Calcutta auction, or simply "Calcutta," is a gambling format used often in golf tournaments. You can use it for a Workout War just to make the game more interesting for those who want to wager more money. Let's say you chose a team competition format with three guys per team, randomly selected, and there are ten teams. The Calcutta is like holding an auction to buy the team you think is going to win the whole competition. Let's say you think Bob, Joe, and Fred are going to be the winning team, so there is an auction, which goes to the highest bidder. You paid $100 for that team. If they win, you earn 70 percent of all the auction money collected for all the teams; second place gets 30 percent of the auction money. Once teams are bought, you can also give the teams the option of buying half of their own team from the person who bought them. So it's like placing a bet on yourself to win.

**Teams with a draft:** Another fun twist for team competition is to incorporate a draft just like in fantasy football. Get the guys together for one last beer, pick two captains, and have them choose up teams.

# SELECT A SCORING METHOD

I already mentioned some of the different ways you can measure results and determine a winner, but let's go through them in more detail.

**Pound-for-pound (actual weight lost):** Nothing fancy here; whoever loses the most weight in pounds at the end of 60 days wins.

**Body-weight percentage lost:** Take the starting body weight and divide it by the actual number of pounds lost, and that will give you the percentage of body weight lost. Example: Chuck weighs 230 pounds at the start of the competition. He loses a total of 25 pounds over the 60-day contest. So you take his starting weight and divide that by total pounds lost—230 / 25 = 9.2. So Chuck lost 9.2 percent of his body weight.

**Body-fat percentage lost:** Everyone starts by measuring their starting body-fat percentage. An independent judge records these figures and keeps them until the end of the competition. After 60 days, everyone measures their ending body-fat percentage. Subtract the ending body-fat percentage from the starting body-fat percentage and you get the total body-fat percentage lost. Highest wins. So if someone starts at 28 percent body fat and ends at 20 percent body fat, he's lost 8 percent body fat. If you don't know how to administer a body-fat test, you might want to enlist the help of a local fitness professional to test and track the results.

**Rival challenges, best times/score:** You can throw a Rival Strength Challenge workout time/score into the competition, too. This refers to one of the key workouts in the program detailed in Part III, which is a timed workout. For example, using the B-52 Bomber workout, you would have all the members of one team do the workout, record their times, and add them up; the other team would then do the same. Whichever team is faster wins. This could count for a bonus 5 pounds of weight subtracted from the final weigh-in for the winning team, or you can come up with whatever incentives you want—get creative. Or if it's a bracket elimination, you could have guys go head-to-head with the rival workout and the winner gets a few-pound advantage at the weigh-in.

**The Combo Deal: percentage of weight and body fat lost:** To keep the playing field as level as possible for all body types, I suggest doing either percentage of weight lost or percentage of body fat lost. Or do what we did for the book's focus group, the Combo Deal. You take the percentage of total weight lost number, as described above, and add that number to the body-fat percentage lost, as described above. The person with the highest sum is the winner. Example: Let's say Bruce was 200 pounds with 25 percent body fat. His final weight is 180 with 18 percent body fat. So his percentage of total weight lost is 10, and his body-fat percentage lost is 7. His total number is 17.

# FIGURE OUT THE DETAILS

Okay, so you've decided what type of competition you want to organize and how it will be judged. Good. You've already scouted out potential players and maybe even started doing some recruiting using the hints suggested in the last chapter. Signing up players will be a lot easier if you have all of the details of the competition ironed out, including kickoff date, rules, and prizes.

Set a tentative start date and give yourself a couple of weeks to recruit players. Once you get a field of competitors together, select an official start date and ending weigh-in 60 days later, give or take a few days.

## SET THE PARAMETERS OF THE COMPETITION

Here's what you need to figure out prior to signing up players:

- Decide on an entry fee or contest buy-in amount.
- Place a cap, if any, on the number of competitors.
- Set teams and brackets.
- Choose prizes for the winner and loser. Ever since we played T-ball or flag football, we couldn't wait until the end of the season so we could get our hands on that trophy. It didn't matter how badly we might have played. Whether we were in first place or last, we knew we were going home with some hardware. We're no different today; we're still that 7-year-old boy yearning to compete and collect a prize. Here are some ideas for prizes:

  - ○ *Trophy or plaque*
  - ○ *Pro wrestling championship toy belt*
  - ○ *Apple-shaped trophy*
  - ○ *Big cup trophy*
  - ○ *Bodybuilder trophy*
  - ○ *Funny plaque*

*Everyone wants a trophy!*

The real motivator, you know, is going to be CASH, GREEN-BACKS, CRISP BENJAMINS! If you want to get your friends on board, bet on weight loss.

Now, you might be asking yourself, "If I collect money, isn't that gambling?" No, not according to the legal definition of gambling: "A person engages in gambling if he stakes or risks something of value upon the outcome of a contest of chance or a future contingent event *not under his control or influence*."

In other words, it's gambling if it entails betting on something beyond your control or influence, like a roulette wheel, a Thorough-

## Prize or Punishment for the Loser

Oh, how we love chuckling at someone else's pain and disappointment. When it comes to pounding someone's face in loser pie, we're the first ones in line. We can't just let them lose and live in peace—no way. They've earned their shame, and now they need to be put on display for the whole world to see. It's all in good fun. So be ruthless.

Here are some gift ideas for the chump or chumps who lose:

**A T-shirt that says . . .**
- I haven't seen my feet since 1983!
- Everybody loves a fat guy
- I beat anorexia
- I'm a fat, hairy loser

**Loser trophy/award:**
- Toilet-seat trophy
- Pig trophy
- Doughnut trophy
- Loser cup
- Donkey-butt trophy

*Make it FUN!*

**Or make the loser award a punishment . . .**
- Loser has to carry his lunch in a Hulk lunch box for a week.
- Loser has to park two or more blocks away from work every week for a month so he gets extra exercise.
- Loser must wear yoga tights to the gym for a week.
- Loser cooks (or buys) dinner for the group.

bred, or the Packers covering the spread this Sunday. When someone puts money on the line in a Workout War competition, he is betting on something that's within his control: his weight (our weight is technically under our control) and fitness level. Thus it's skill based and, in the eyes of the law, not gambling. This is one of the main reasons why diet-betting Web sites are springing up, fast and furious, all over the Internet.

That said, if you are going to be running this out of your office, check with your supervisor first, as you would with any other office pool. Once you get the okay, take his or her money, too!

## CONSIDER DONATING THE WINNINGS TO CHARITY

Cash contests can also be great opportunities to turn your fun and fitness into help for others. Consider donating the money payout to a charity. If you like this idea, you have some decisions to make. Will it be a preselected charity? Will the money be donated in the winner's name or will the winner be able to choose his favorite charity?

## PICK A BANKER TO HANDLE THE FUNDS

It's best to use an outsider, a nonplayer with no ties to the competition. He or she will hold and distribute the money after the game is over.

## ASSIGN A REFEREE

As with football pools, this is a commissioner of sorts who will make final decisions when something is in question. Referees can also make sure that the rules are followed for weigh-ins, such as taking legitimate weigh-in photos. It's a good idea to make this someone who has no ties to the game or its players.

## FIGURE OUT THE WEIGH-INS

What method will you use to take and track results? Will you have weekly in-person weigh-ins? Will you use a third party to do weigh-ins (fitness center, doctor's office, CVS Minute Clinic, etc.)? If your participants are scattered across town or across the country, you may require participants to take photos of themselves standing on a scale holding the daily newspaper so everyone can see the date.

## ESTABLISH AN ONLINE HUB

Think of it as a virtual water cooler where combatants gather to trash talk, record their stats, and check rankings on a leaderboard.

# Keeping It Legit: Best Practices for a Fair Contest

Well-run weight-loss contests have strictly organized measurement events. Doing it right lends legitimacy to the whole deal and motivates contestants to take it seriously. Here are some tips for making weigh-ins and body-fat analysis top-notch.

## Weigh-Ins

1. Bring a digital scale to a preselected location and have all the participants weigh in at the same time and place.
2. Do a weigh-in at a third-party location such as CVS Minute Clinic, Walgreens, a doctor's office, or with a preselected personal trainer or fitness center. Some of these may include fees for service.
3. Long-distance contestants: Have participants who can't travel to the weigh-in take a photo of themselves on the scale and send it digitally to the referee. Make sure that they hold something showing the date the photo was taken, such as a newspaper.

## Body-Fat Testing

1. Hire a personal trainer or weight-loss center to administer the test. You can have the trainer do the weigh-in and body-fat test at the same time.
2. Use body-fat calipers over electronic handheld versions. The electronic ones are not nearly as accurate.

Choose an impartial referee to administer the measurements

**Weekly weigh-in:** If it's a local group or group of coworkers, a weekly weigh-in could really keep the guys on task and promote lots and lots of trash talking.

**Trash talk:** The trash talking always is best when done face-to-face, but anything will do—group text messages, group e-mails, social media groups. Most of the time, it's not necessarily the leader bragging; it's guys ripping on the dudes who are in last place.

**Leaderboards:** A leaderboard is great so guys can see where they stand and see if they need to step it up. It could be just a simple body-weight graph or chart on a Facebook community page that shows where each competitor is, or if it's a team competition, each team could see who is winning.

If you prefer to use another system, there are many online tracking Web sites that can help you host a weight-loss challenge. One of the better ones is DietBet.com, which provides an easy forum for tracking and collecting money, communicating, and paying out winnings. Go to DietBet.com to start your own contest or jump into one that's already organized and about to start. Follow the simple instructions on how to set it up, and DietBet takes care of the rest. With this site you can run challenges with two to fifty players. They collect the money for you and send out e-mails to your players. You can stay in contact with your players through the DietBet Web site and iPhone app.

Here are some other fitness competition sites to consider:

- FitFeud.com
- Skinnyo.com
- Thintopia.com
- Fatbet.net
- WeightLossWars.com
- HealthyWage.com

## CRANK IT UP

Start building buzz and getting the ball rolling.

- Send out reminder e-mails.
- Collect entry fees. Send an e-mail to those who have paid or not paid as a receipt. Establish a cutoff date for people to pay the entry fee.
- Set up a community bulletin board online or use the MensHealth/WorkoutWar.com forums.
- Kick off the contest with an official weigh-in, clarify rules, and answer questions. Pick the exact time, place, and date to do the official weigh-in; you could hand out copies of the official rules, collect any entry fees that have not been collected, and answer any questions that people may have. The rules should be clear before people show up, but there will probably be some last-minute contestants wanting to join in, depending on what type of contest you are hosting.

Let the trash talking begin!

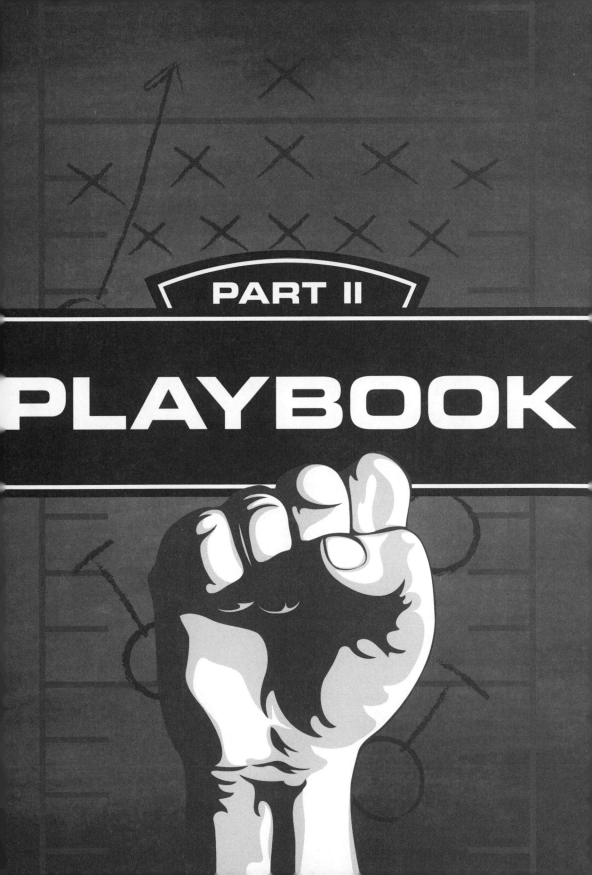

PART II

# PLAYBOOK

# SWEAT TO WIN

④

## THE WORKOUT WARRIOR'S MUSCLE-UP PLAN

**HAVE YOU EVER WONDERED WHAT IT TAKES PHYSICALLY AND MENTALLY TO REALLY TRAIN LIKE A WORLD CHAMPION ATHLETE?** Well, you're about to find out. In my years as a professional strength and conditioning coach, I have noticed that all champions have several things in common.

- They are committed.
- They have a plan.
- They are goal oriented.
- They train hard in the weight room, so they can play harder.
- They have a no-excuses attitude.
- They are leaders.
- They believe in themselves almost to the point of being cocky.

# "RULE #76: NO EXCUSES, PLAY LIKE A CHAMPION."

—VINCE VAUGHN IN *WEDDING CRASHERS*

If you want to be a world champion, you have to adopt this kind of attitude. Champions do the work in the weight room so they will excel on the court or field on game day. I have done all that I can to ensure your success by programming a world-class training schedule while laying the plan out so it's so easy that a Neanderthal could follow it.

If you follow this plan, your body will change. If you sandbag your workouts, you will fail. If you skip workouts, you will lose. The choice is yours.

To ensure the best results, these workouts are based on science and research, so you need to follow them as prescribed. You will always start off any workout with a proper warmup you can do on your own. However, I highly suggest that you do the warmup routine on page 47.

## THE WARRIOR'S WORKOUTS

To recap your personal game plan: This is a 60-day program made up of four 12-day quarters and an "OT," an overtime period. The workouts (and eating plans) change for every segment of the 2-month challenge. *You will exercise every day,* that is, if you want to win.

Each 12-day quarter contains four types of workouts, which you will cycle through. Here's a snapshot of them:

**Rival Strength Challenges:** This workout is fast paced and will tax your muscular endurance and strength. It's you against the clock and your friends, and you will go to muscular failure or close to it if you push yourself. These workouts will burn a ton of calories because your heart rate will be elevated for the entire workout. Post your time after finishing your workout and see if you can beat that time when doing that workout again. Or see if the other players can beat your time.

**Functional Stability Workouts:** This is a noncardiovascular type of workout consisting of functional movements that will strengthen your core, increase flexibility, and work the areas that are often neglected in other types of workouts. These programs will enhance performance but will also increase your chances of remaining injury free. Functional strength training develops and strengthens the stabilizing muscles necessary to perform everyday and athletic movements.

**HIIT Workouts:** HIIT stands for high-intensity interval training, a specialized form of interval training that involves short bouts of maximum-intensity exercise, separated by rest intervals or low-intensity exercise. These workouts will challenge your body while decreasing the chance of plateaus, boredom, or dropping out. HIIT causes metabolic adaptations that enable you to use more fat as fuel under a variety of conditions. You will burn a high number of calories during these workouts and after because your metabolism will stay elevated long after you hit the showers.

**Cardio Workouts:** These are pretty straightforward. On cardio days, you'll perform any cardiovascular exercise of your choosing, such as power walking, hiking, running (on a treadmill, road, or trail), lap swimming, inline skating, golfing (walk the course), friendly basketball, handball, tennis, pool jogging, canoeing, kayaking, bike riding (stationary or outdoor), or taking a group fitness class.

The rules for your cardio workouts are simple:

● Make sure to warm up properly. If you can't hold a conversation, you're working too hard.

- You should always work between 60 and 80 percent of your maximum heart rate or a 6 to 8 on the RPE (rate of perceived exertion) scale.

- Activities should last NO less than 20 minutes. As you progress through the program, your cardio sessions will last longer.

I designed the workouts to get progressively harder over the course of the quarters and overtime. However, your current fitness level will dictate how hard you should be working during each phase. Choose a workout level to fit your current needs, not the needs of when you were playing college ball. See the RPE (Rate of Perceived Exertion) scale cheat sheet on page 45 to learn how to gauge and change your effort. As you cycle through the next 60 days, your body will adapt and let you know if you can handle more.

The Rival Strength Challenge days are the meat and potatoes of all the workouts and have names like B-52 Bomber and 747. This way you can refer to the workouts by name when you're taunting your competition and comparing results.

All the workouts use either your body weight or a single pair of dumbbells for resistance. This way you don't have to join an expensive health club or turn your house into a gym. If you travel for a living or have a small living space, you will still be able to perform the entire workout as intended.

Now, before you jump in with both feet, let's establish a baseline and create some clear goals. On any journey, you need to know where you want to go, and you have to know where you're starting. That's the purpose of the next step, called The Combine.

## THE COMBINE

A "combine" in football and basketball, as you know, is an event where prospective players show off their bodies and their skills to team recruiters and coaches. It gives scouts a baseline to judge prospective draftees against one another when they are trying to flesh out their lineups and rosters. Here, we're going to use a combine approach to help you establish a baseline of fitness and record your physiological goals. Grab a sheet of paper or a computer or use the space below to log some basic data.

## STARTING STATS

Starting weight: _____pounds

Starting body-fat composition: _____ %

Goal weight and/or body fat:_____ pounds/%

(You will most likely need a fitness professional to administer the body-fat percentage test for you, or you can use an electronic hand-held device or calipers. Note that calipers, a means of pinching the body fat, are more reliable than the electronic handheld devices.)

Starting fitness score: _____(See test below.)

Goals: _____

_____

_____

_____

_____

# THE HOW-FIT-ARE-YOU TEST

You think you're a gamer, but how fit are you, really? A simple test of three body-weight exercises will accurately evaluate your fitness level and probably issue you a significant wake-up call. To do the test, you will need to wear loose-fitting workout clothes and running shoes. You'll also need:

- An open space
- A timer set to go off at 10 minutes
- A piece of paper or some way of counting/marking down your rounds

# LEGENDS:
## The Making of a Champion

# SHAQUILLE O'NEAL
### aka "The Diesel"

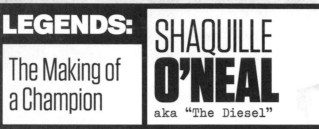

When Shaq was in his prime and dominating guys in the paint, he knew that keeping his legs and core strong and powerful was a key ingredient to his success. Nobody in the league could hold their ground on him in the post.

Shaq loved to make his workouts fun by pumping up the music as loud as possible and, of course, talking some smack. Sometimes he would challenge a teammate to see how far they could throw the heaviest medicine ball, or who could rep out 500 pounds on the leg press the most times. (Shaq once did 1,200 pounds on the leg press 15 times.) It was all about making working out fun and challenging, while getting results on the court.

One of his favorite exercises was using a jumping machine that we had when I was the strength coach for the Lakers. This machine would record how much power you could produce on every jump. Shaq and power forward Mark "Mad Dog" Madsen loved to go head–to–head on this machine all the time, kind of like a Rival Strength Challenge. Find a similar way to add more competitiveness to your own workouts.

# THE TEST

Hold on. Before you go nuts, warm up your muscles. I suggest using the body-weight warmup recommended in the next chapter, which includes doing squats, toe touches, arm circles, jumping jacks, hip circles, side lunge stretches, and spiderman lunge stretches to both sides. That'll do the trick.

| COMPLETED ROUNDS | YOUR SCORE |
|------------------|------------|
| 4 or less | Benchwarmer |
| 5 to 7 | Junior Varsity |
| 8 to 10 | Varsity |
| 11+ | All-Star |

Take a rest. Then, when you are ready, hit your stopwatch or timer and begin exercising: Perform 5 burpees, 10 pushups, and 15 squats one after the other. (Note: Don't add a pushup to the burpee movement.) Once you get through all three exercises, that counts as one round (take note). Then start over. See how many rounds you can complete in 10 minutes. You must finish all 15 squats for it to count as a complete round. Rest when you need to, but it's only 10 minutes, so push yourself. When the timer goes off, record your number of completed rounds on a sheet of paper and compare it to the key above.

At the end of the contest, around day 60, weigh and measure yourself and retake the fitness test. Record your scores below.

## ENDING STATS (DAY 61 CHECK-IN)

Ending weight: _____ pounds

Total pounds lost:_____ pounds

Ending body-fat percentage: _____ %

Total body-fat percentage lost:_____ %

Ending fitness score:_____

# LAST-MINUTE WORKOUT TIPS AND ADVICE

Before you start sampling the exercises in the next chapter and jump into the kickoff in the first quarter, keep this advice in mind to get the most out of your workouts:

- Be well rested. You need to sleep in order to have energy to push yourself hard enough during your workouts. Remember that sleep is when your body produces growth hormone and when your muscles repair. Cheat sleep and you cheat muscle growth.

- Blast the tunes! Research has shown that music that motivates you can enhance your performance.

- Work out with a buddy. Feed off each other's energy and challenge one another to push harder.

- Change the location of your workout. Tired of exercising in your man cave? Take it outside. Changing locations can help raise your energy and motivation level.

- Read back over any trash talk posted by your friends. Use those words as fuel to crush them. Winning is sweet revenge.

- Monitor the level of your effort. It's real easy to have a down day and slack on your workout. So how do you know if you're just going through the motions or if you're working hard enough to make a difference?

    If you have a heart rate monitor, by all means use it! However, if you don't have one and getting one that tracks your calorie burn just isn't in the budget, there is a fairly easy-to-use system called the Borg Rate of Perceived Exertion Scale (RPE). Although subjective, it tends to be fairly accurate. RPE is a way of internally scanning your body and assessing how hard it's working based on the following: increased heart rate, muscle fatigue, amount of perspiration, and any dizziness or nausea you may be experiencing. At any time during your workout, ask yourself, "How hard am I working? Can I push harder or do I need to ease off the gas a little?" Take a look at the exertion levels I've adapted from the Borg RPE in the cheat sheet opposite. For your workouts, you'll want to stay somewhere in the vicinity of 6 and 8. No matter what these idiots on television tell you, puking is not a badge of honor. Nausea and dizziness are your body telling you, "Hey, idiot, back off, you're killing me." If this happens, step off the gas (intensity) and allow your workout intensity to build back up gradually.

# RPE SCALE CHEAT SHEET

| RATING | EXERTION LEVEL |
|--------|----------------|
| 0 | Nothing. You're laid up in the La-Z-Boy watching the game, shoveling chips into your trap. |
| 1 | Almost nothing. Doing the dishes to earn brownie points with your lady. |
| 2 | Very, very light. You're walking to the mailbox. |
| 3 | Fairly light. You're using a push mower to mow a small lawn. |
| 4 | Light. Riding a bike around the block with your kids. |
| 5 | Moderate. Now you're exercising! |
| 6 | Fairly hard. Your heart rate is climbing and your muscles are warmed up and starting to burn. |
| 7 | Hard. Now you're starting to leave the competition in the dust. Sweat is pouring off your brow and your muscles feel like they could explode. |
| 8 | Very hard. You are sucking wind, almost to your limit, but you're hanging on. |
| 9 | Extremely hard. Starting to see stars. You don't know how much longer you can hang on. |
| 10 | Beyond hard. Gonna puke! The room is spinning! |

# THE EXERCISES

## THIS IS WHERE THE MUSCLE IS MADE!

**THERE ARE ABOUT AS MANY WAYS TO EXERCISE AS THERE ARE TRAINERS WHO THINK THEIR WAY IS THE BEST.** In all honesty, you can win your competition using any diet and exercise routine you like as long as the combo leaves you with a calorie deficit at the end of the day, and the training is tough enough to burn fat and build muscle. So if you have a favorite workout, go for it. If you need some instruction and a solid program that doesn't require a lot of gear, then you've come to the right place. On the following pages, you'll find photos and descriptions of metabolic moves and strength exercises that will fit nicely into your competition game plan. Be sure to begin every workout with a warmup of 10 repetitions of squats, toe touches, arm circles, jumping jacks, hip circles, side lunge stretches, and spiderman lunge stretches.

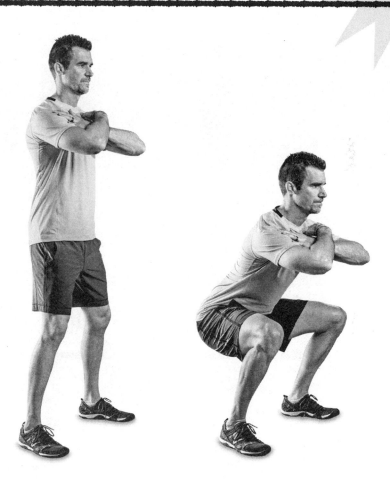

## SQUAT

Stand with your feet shoulder-width apart or slightly wider, arms crossed in front of your chest with hands touching your shoulders. Begin by pushing your hips and butt back while bending the knees. Squat until the tops of your thighs are parallel to the ground and then push through your heels to return to the starting position. Try to keep your back straight, chest up, and head looking straight ahead. Don't let the knees push out past the toes. Do the prescribed number of reps.

*If you have trouble with the knees going forward or you can't squat down far enough, try elevating your heels about an inch off the ground by standing on an inch-high board or weight plates and extend your arms straight out in front of you.

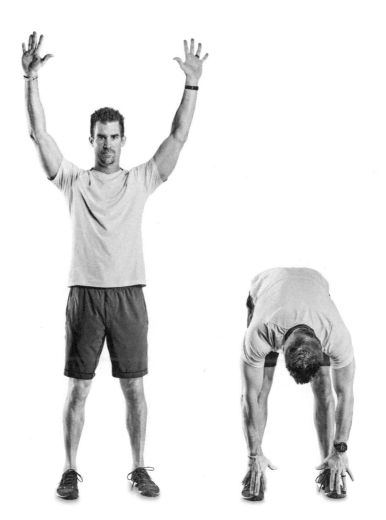

## TOE TOUCH

Stand with your feet shoulder-width apart and your arms extended overhead toward the ceiling. With a slight bend in the knees, hinge forward from the hips and try to touch your fingers to your toes, feeling a stretch in your hamstrings. Hold for only one second and then stand back up to the starting position with arms reaching toward the ceiling. Repeat for the prescribed number of reps.

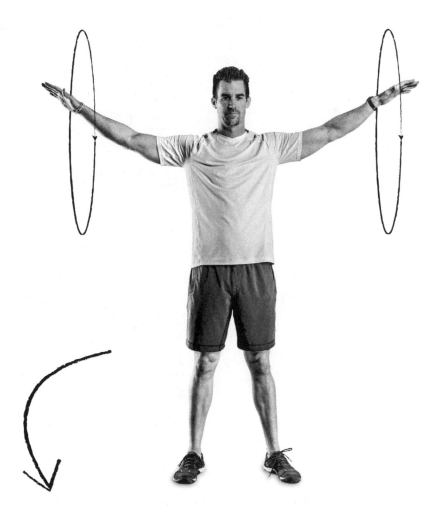

# ARM CIRCLE

Stand with your arms out to your sides at shoulder height, palms down. Perform a forward circle with both arms at the same time. Do 10 circles forward and then repeat the same 10 circles backward.

# JUMPING JACK

Stand with your feet close together and arms by your sides. Simultaneously jump your feet out and bring the hands up to at least shoulder height, then jump the feet back and lower your arms to the starting position. Repeat this movement rapidly for the prescribed time or reps.

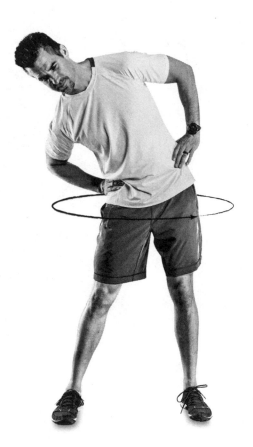

# HIP CIRCLE

Stand with your feet about shoulder-width apart and place your hands on your hips. Make a circle with your hips, swaying out and around while your upper body tilts slightly in the direction opposite of your hips for balance. Perform 10 circles in one direction and then perform 10 circles in the other direction.

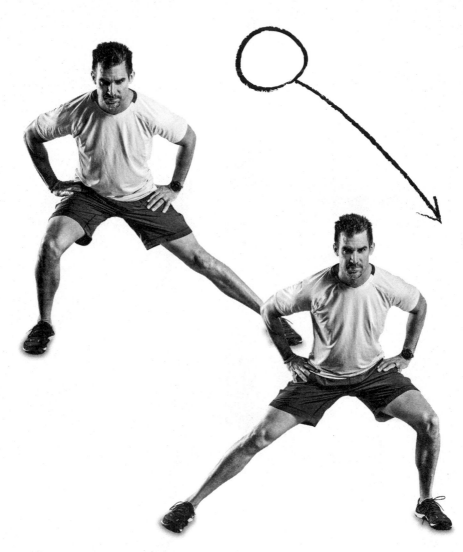

## SIDE LUNGE STRETCH

Start with your feet wider than shoulder-width apart, feet facing forward. Take a big step laterally to the right with your right foot, keeping your left foot planted on the floor. Bend your right knee to 90 degrees to sink into the lunge while keeping your left leg straight. Avoid bouncing into the lunge and be careful that your right knee does not move forward of your right foot's toes. Hold this position for a second and then press off your right foot to straighten back into the standing position. Repeat, this time stepping laterally with your left foot. That's one rep. Continue lunging from side to side for a total of 10 reps, pausing a second each time.

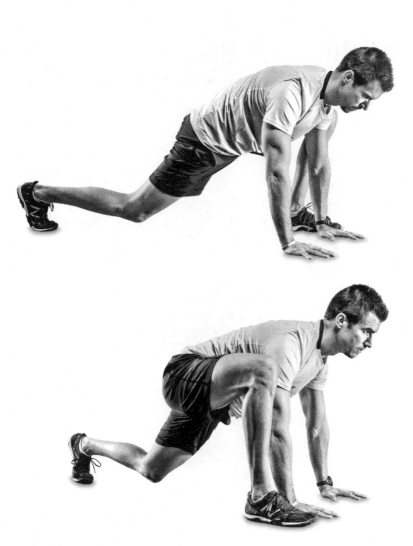

# SPIDERMAN LUNGE STRETCH

Assume a pushup position with your body suspended between your hands and toes. Your hands should be directly under your shoulders. Now, lift your left foot and bring it toward your left hand or, if possible, place it just outside your left hand. Your right leg stays extended behind you. (Beginners should go halfway between the arm and the waist. As mobility increases, move the foot up to the hand.) Hold this position for five seconds. Return to the starting position and stretch the right leg forward. That's one rep. Continue alternating legs for 10 reps.

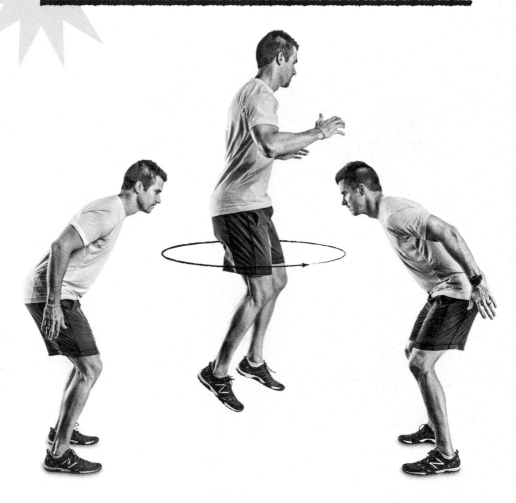

## 180 JUMP

Stand with your feet shoulder-width apart. Squat down into a half-squat position and then jump explosively, rotating your body 180 degrees while in the air. You'll land facing behind where you started. Upon landing under control, dip into another half squat and then jump explosively again, rotating in the other direction back to the starting position. So if you rotate left to start, you will rotate right back to the start. That is one repetition. Continue this movement back and forth for the prescribed reps or time.

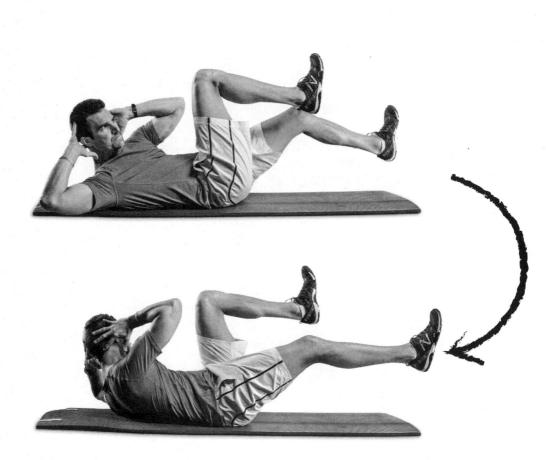

## BICYCLE CRUNCH

Lie on your back with your hands behind your head. Elevate your legs off the floor so both knees are bent at 90 degrees. Press your lower back into the floor, curl your upper back off the floor, and tighten your abdominal muscles. Simultaneously move your left elbow and right knee toward each other while straightening your left leg (don't let it touch the ground). Then bring your left knee back up and immediately move your right elbow and left knee toward each other while straightening your right leg. That's one rep. Do the prescribed number of reps.

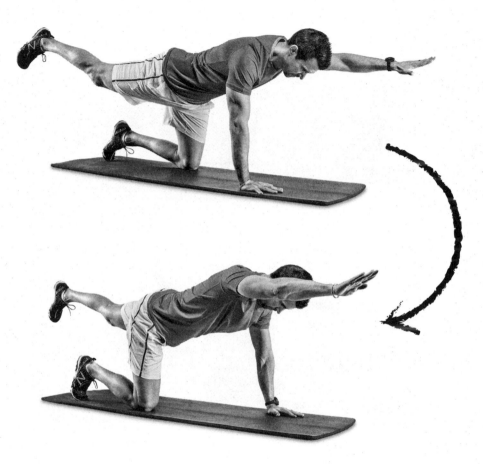

# BIRD DOG

Start on all fours with your hands under your shoulders and knees under hips. Keeping your back flat, simultaneously extend your right leg behind you and your left arm in front of you so both are parallel with the floor. Hold this position for a second and then return your knee and hand to the floor. Next, fully extend your left leg and right arm so they are parallel with the floor. That's one rep. Make sure the spine stays neutral throughout the movement. Do the prescribed number of reps.

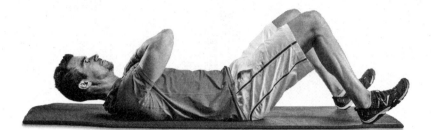

# CRUNCH

Lie on your back with knees bent and heels on the floor. Cross your arms over your chest and place your hands on your shoulders. Curl your upper back off the floor and tighten your stomach muscles. Hold for one second and then return under control back to the starting position. That's one rep. Do the prescribed number of reps.

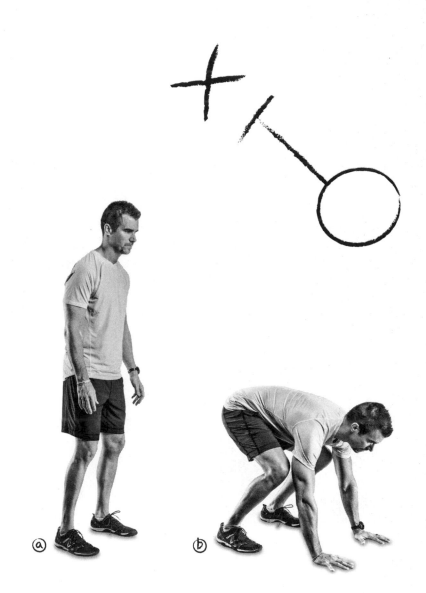

## BURPEE

Stand with your feet about shoulder-width apart (a). Bend your knees to squat and bring your hands to the floor in front of your feet (b). Jump your feet back into a pushup position with your arms straight (c). Then jump your feet back toward your hands and from this crouched position (d), press

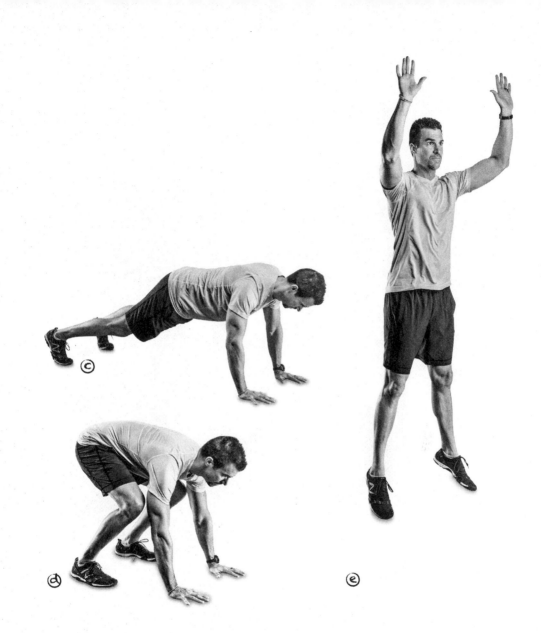

your feet into the floor and swing your arms up to jump explosively so your feet come off the floor (e). Land on the balls of your feet with soft knees and immediately squat again to do another burpee. This movement is performed as rapidly as possible while keeping good form. Do as many as prescribed. You can make it even more challenging by adding a pushup before jumping your feet back.

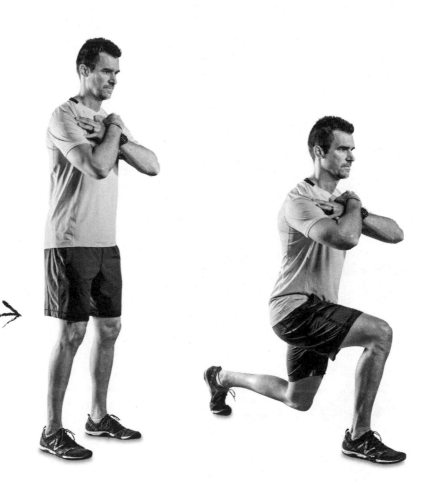

# FORWARD LUNGE

Stand with your feet hip-width apart, arms crossed with fingers touching shoulders, abs tight. Step forward, placing your foot on the ground with your weight evenly distributed on the foot. As the foot lands, make sure to evenly distribute your weight on that foot and begin to lower your hips/body toward the ground, bending both knees. Lower until your front thigh is parallel to the ground, but do not touch the back knee to the ground. Then firmly push off that front leg to return to the starting position. Repeat by stepping forward with the opposite foot. That's one rep. Make sure to keep your upper body upright in good posture and step out far enough so that the front knee stays over the foot in the lunge position. Do the prescribed number of reps.

*Do not let your front knee extend out past your front toes.

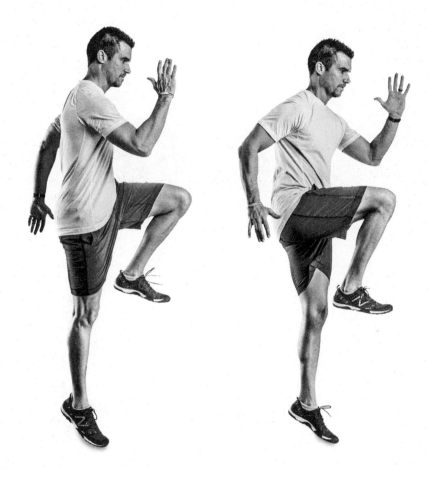

# HIGH KNEE

Stand with your feet together. Now pull one knee up in front of you and bring the opposite arm up as if you are running and then rapidly bring the other knee and arm up as you are bringing the starting knee down. This is just like running in place except that you exaggerate the knee lift, bringing it as high as possible. Perform rapidly and continuously for the prescribed time or reps.

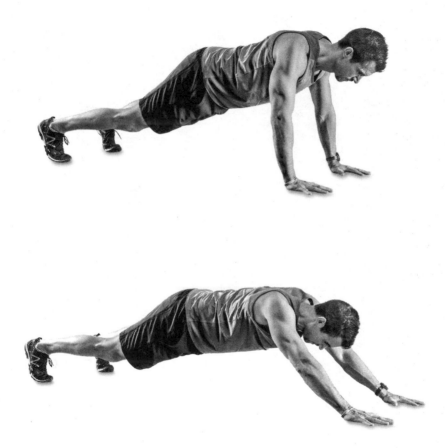

## INCHWORM, HAND WALKOUT

Assume a pushup position with your hands on the floor under your shoulders, arms straight. Keeping your back straight and abs tight, walk your hands out in front of you in small (inchworm-style) steps as far as you can and then inchworm your way back to the starting position. That's one rep. If this move is too difficult, regress it by doing it from a modified pushup position with your knees on the floor. Do the prescribed number of reps.

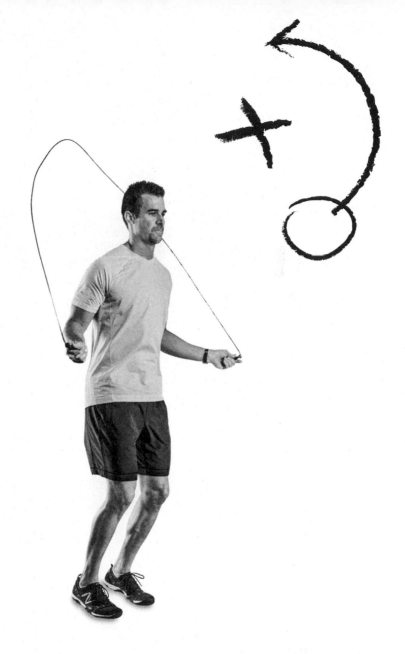

# JUMP ROPE

With feet hip-width apart, jump up and down on the balls of your feet as you swing the rope over you. If you don't have a jump rope, pretend you have an imaginary jump rope. Perform for the required time or reps.

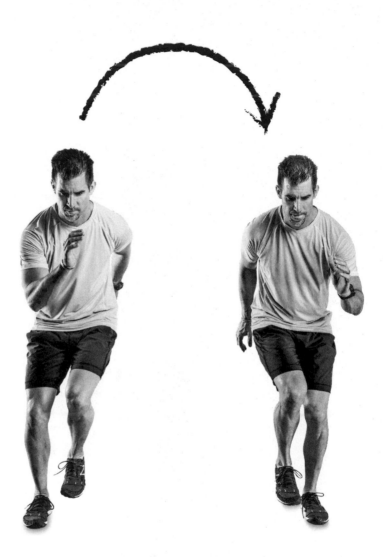

# LATERAL BOUND

Stand with your feet close together and knees slightly bent. Push off your right foot while lifting the left foot off the floor and bound sideways through the air, landing on the left foot. Stick the landing for a second and then push back in the other direction, landing on the right foot. That's one rep. Continue bounding back and forth, maintaining balance and control with each leap. Increase the speed and distance as you become better at this movement. Do the prescribed number of reps.

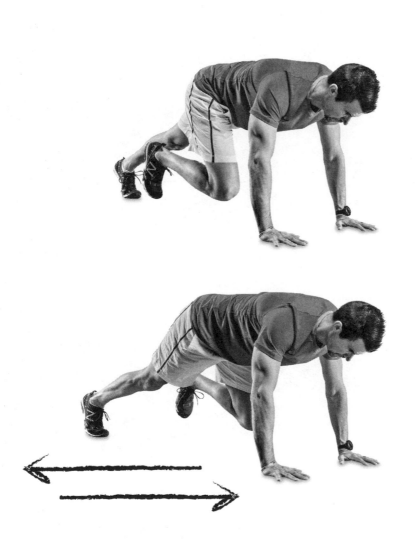

# MOUNTAIN CLIMBER

Assume a plank position by placing your hands on the floor slightly wider than shoulder-width apart and supporting yourself on the balls of your feet. Your arms should be straight. Now, position one leg forward bent under your body; this is the starting position. Keeping your upper body stable and back flat, alternate the leg positions rapidly, landing on the balls of the feet simultaneously. Each leg up and back is one repetition. Do the prescribed number of reps.

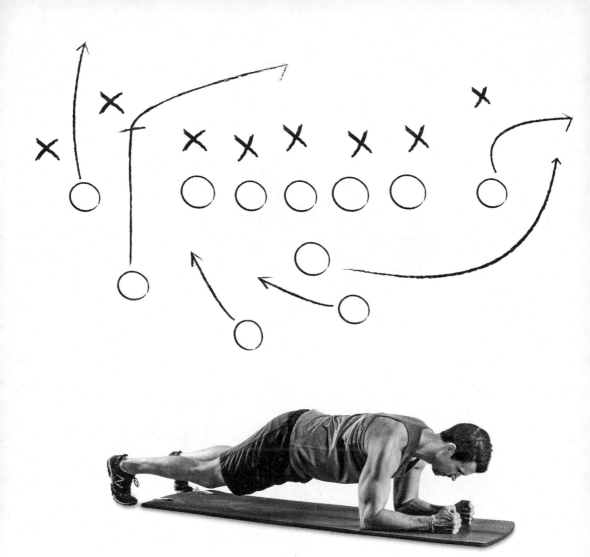

## PLANK

Get into a pushup position with feet hip-width apart and then bend your elbows 90 degrees and support your weight with your forearms on the floor. Your elbows should be directly beneath your shoulders, and your body should form a straight line from your head to your heels. Hold this position for the prescribed amount of time.

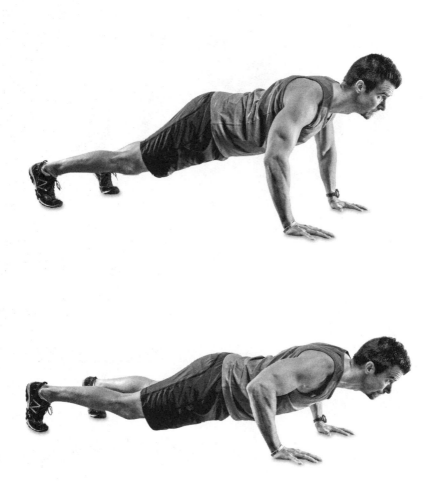

# PUSHUP

Start in the pushup position with your hands on the floor so they're slightly more than shoulder-width apart. Your fingers should point forward. Rise up onto your toes so that all your weight is on your hands and feet. Engage your abdominals to keep your torso in a straight line from heels to head and prevent arching or rounding your back. Bend your elbows and slowly lower your chest to the floor to where the elbows are bent slightly beyond 90 degrees, then push off the floor explosively so that you return to the starting position. That's one rep. Do the prescribed number of reps.

*If this is too difficult, you can perform the same movement with your hands elevated on a step or bench.

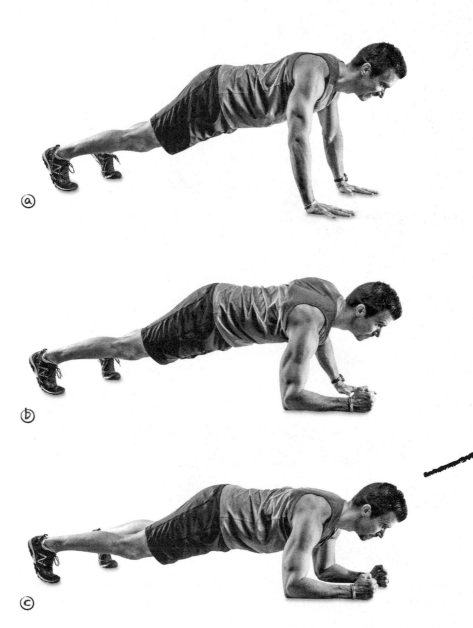

# PLANK PUSHUP

Start in the basic pushup position with your hands directly under your shoulders, arms straight (a). Place your feet a little wider than hip-width apart for greater stability. Keeping your back flat and core engaged, bend one arm 90 degrees and place the forearm on the floor (b). Next, bend the other arm and place its forearm on the floor (c). Now you should be in the forearm

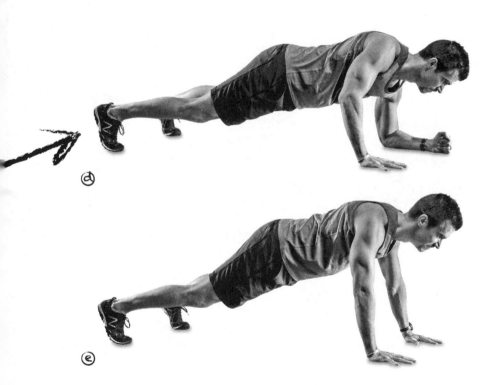

plank position with your body elevated straight between your elbows and the balls of your feet. Pause a second and then press up with one hand at a time (d), until you are back in the original pushup position (e). That's one rep. Repeat for the prescribed number of repetitions.

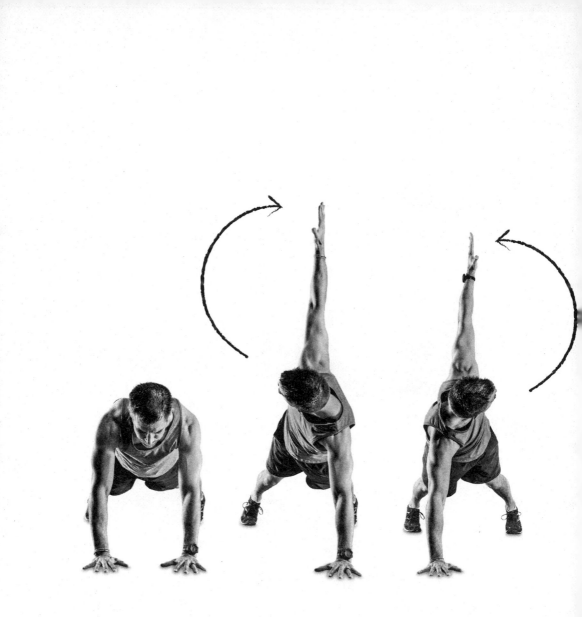

## PUSHUP-POSITION REACHBACK

Start in the pushup position with your arms straight, hands directly under your shoulders. Place the balls of your feet about shoulder width apart for stability. Maintaining stable hips and core, take one arm off the ground and reach back behind you. Turn your head and upper body only and point your arm toward the ceiling. Pause, then return back to the starting position. Repeat with the other arm on the other side. That's one rep. Make sure to keep your hips and core stable throughout the movement. Do the prescribed number of reps.

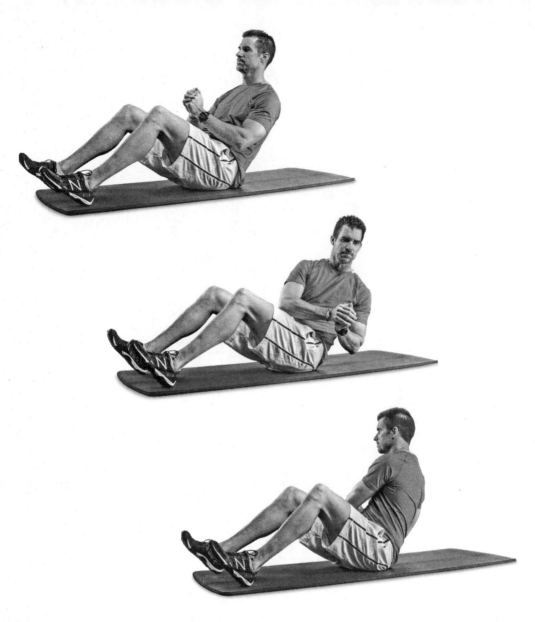

# SEATED RUSSIAN TWIST

Sit on the floor with your hips bent 90 degrees and your heels on the floor, legs bent 45 degrees. Hold a light weight with both hands or clasp your hands together (as shown) in front of you and keep your back straight (your torso should be at about 45 degrees to the floor). At a medium speed, twist your torso as far as you can to the left and then reverse the motion, twisting as far as you can to the right. That's one rep. Do the prescribed number of reps.

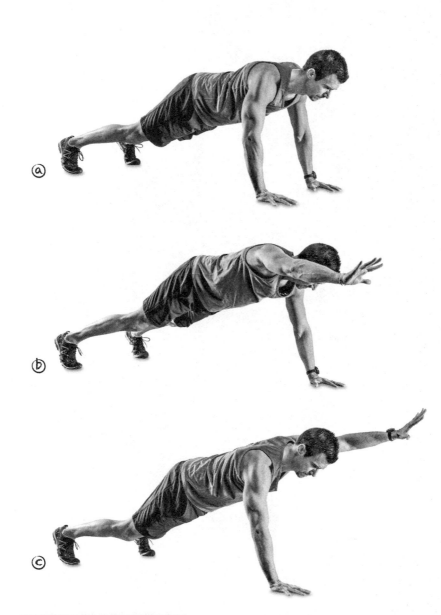

## PUSHUP PLANK MATRIX

Start in the basic pushup position, but spread your feet shoulder-width apart (a); hold this position for 10 seconds, keeping your abdominals tight. Next, lift one arm off the floor, straighten it out in front of you, and hold for 10 seconds, keeping your hips square and level (b), before returning to the starting position. Now lift and straighten your other arm out in front of you (c)

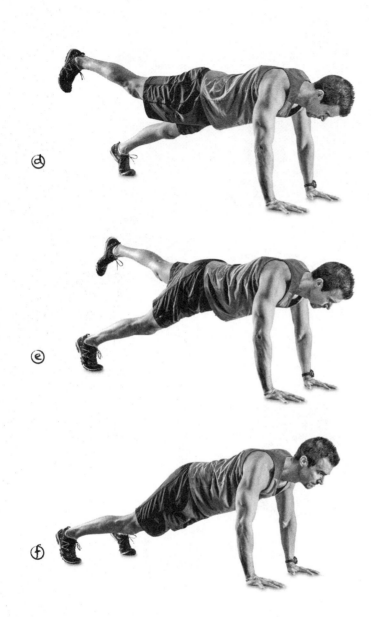

and hold that for 10 seconds before returning to start. Next, lift one leg about 2 feet above the floor and hold for 10 seconds (d). Return that foot to the floor, lift the opposite leg off the floor, and hold for 10 seconds (e). Finally, finish by holding the pushup plank for 10 seconds (f). Total time is 60 seconds.

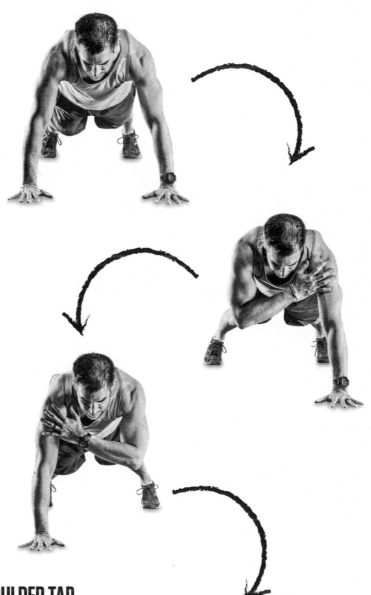

## SHOULDER TAP

Start in the pushup position with arms straight, hands directly under your shoulders. Your feet should be about shoulder-width apart for greater stability. Without dropping or rotating your hips, take your right hand off the floor and tap your left shoulder. Immediately put it back on the floor and then lift your left hand and tap the right shoulder. That's one rep. Keep alternating the shoulder taps while keeping your hips still. Do the prescribed number of reps.

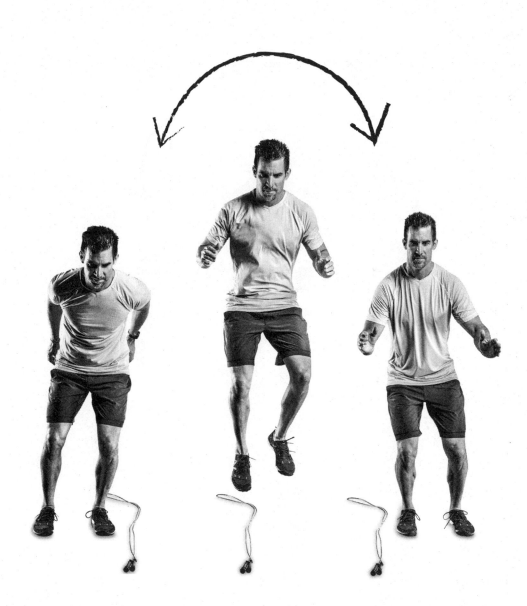

## SIDE-TO-SIDE JUMP

Stand with your feet hip-width apart and knees slightly bent. Place a yardstick or jump rope on the floor to the left of you and jump over it sideways with both feet, landing on both feet at the same time. Quickly jump back to the starting position. Stay on the balls of the feet for the entire time, quickly bouncing back and forth sideways with both feet for the required reps or time.

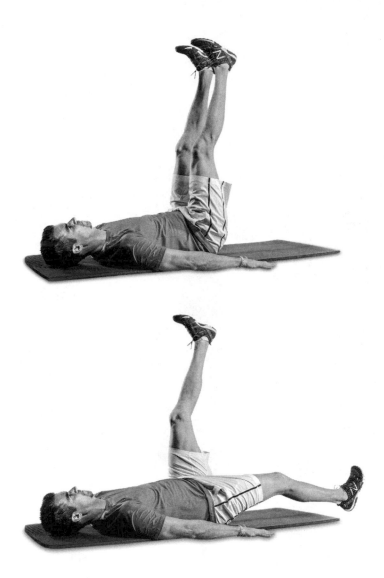

## SINGLE-LEG DROP

Lie flat on your back with your arms on the floor by your sides and raise both legs straight up toward the ceiling. Keeping your lower back pressed into the floor and your abdominals engaged, lower one leg toward the floor (touch the floor if you can) and then bring that leg all the way back up to the starting position. Repeat with the other leg. That's one rep. Do the prescribed number of reps.

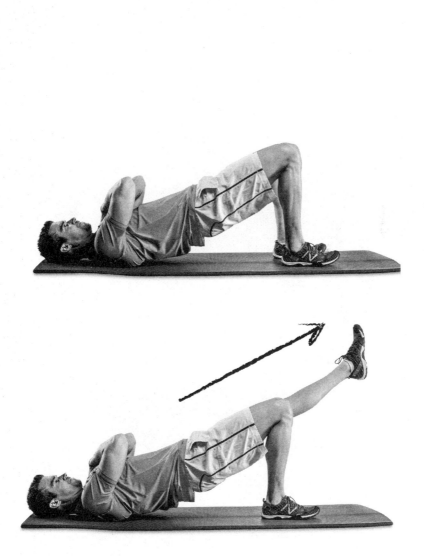

# SINGLE-LEG BRIDGE

Lie on your back with your knees bent and together and your feet together and flat on the floor. Cross your arms over your chest and place each hand on the opposite shoulder. Now squeeze your glutes and raise your hips off the floor. This is the starting position. Keeping your hips level, lift your left leg off the floor and straighten it. Focus on squeezing your right glute. Hold this position for 5 seconds, then bring the left leg back to the floor and repeat using the other leg. That's one rep. Keep switching back and forth for the prescribed reps.

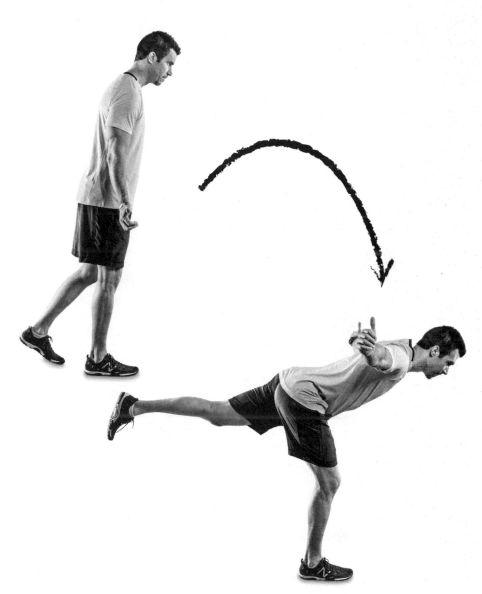

## SINGLE-LEG ROMANIAN DEADLIFT

Standing on one foot with your knee slightly bent, slowly bend forward at the hips while raising your elevated leg behind you. Raise your arms out to your sides (like airplane wings), thumbs up, for balance. Bend forward as far as you can while maintaining that posture until you feel a stretch in your hamstring on the down leg. Then raise your body and lower your leg back to the starting position. Perform all the required reps on one leg, then switch to the other leg.

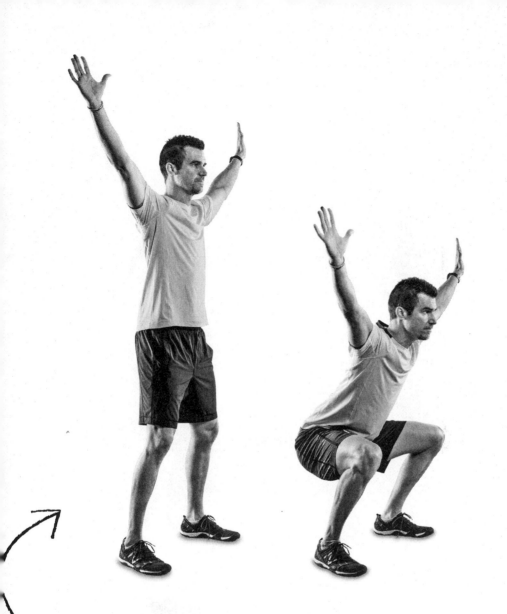

## SQUAT WITH ARMS UP

Stand with your feet shoulder-width apart and raise your arms above your head to make a V. Now push your butt back as if sitting into a chair and bend your legs to squat until your thighs are parallel with the floor or lower. Pause and then press your feet into the floor to straighten your legs. That's one rep. Arms stay overhead throughout the movement. Do the prescribed number of reps.

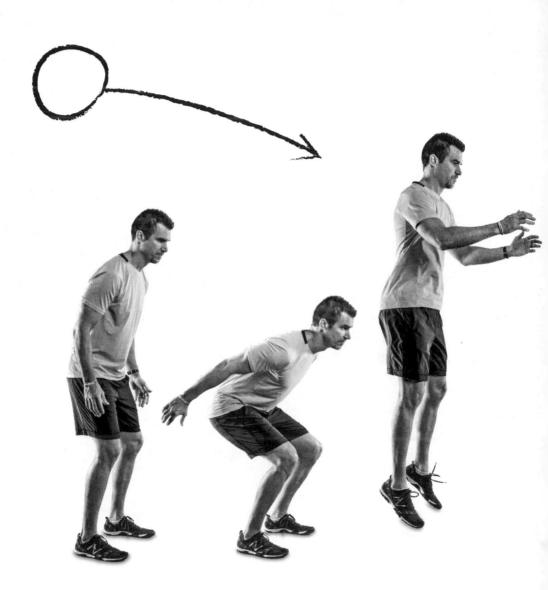

## SQUAT JUMP

Stand with your feet shoulder-width apart or slightly wider, arms hanging by your sides. Begin by pushing your hips and butt back while bending at the knees as you would do in a normal squat. Then quickly press your feet into the floor, straighten your legs, and thrust your hips forward to explosively jump straight up. Land as softly as possible and then quickly go back down into the next squat and jump again. Perform without stopping for the required time or reps.

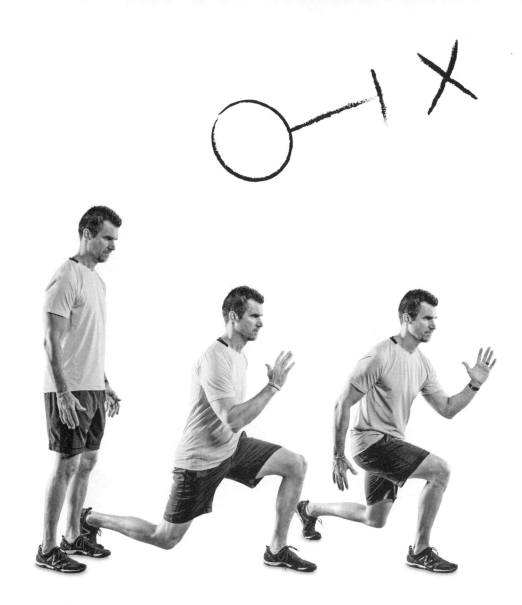

# WALKING LUNGE

Stand with your feet hip-width apart. Take a big step forward with one foot and dip into a forward lunge position until your front thigh is parallel with the floor and your back knee hovers a few inches above the floor. Now, instead of pushing back into the starting position, push up through the front leg and bring the back leg forward to come back to the feet-together position. You will be traveling forward during this exercise, so you will need some space. Next, lunge forward with the opposite foot and continue alternating legs for time or reps.

# DUMBBELL STRENGTH EXERCISES

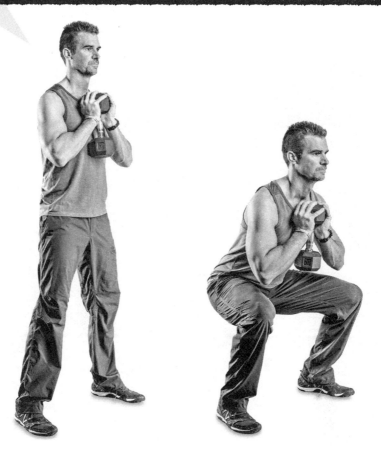

## GOBLET SQUAT

Stand with your feet shoulder-width apart and hold a heavy dumbbell with both hands grasping one end of the dumbbell, not the handle, at chest level. You'll hold the dumbbell vertically so it resembles a goblet. Begin by pushing your hips and butt back while bending at the knees. Squat until the tops of your thighs are parallel to the ground and then push through your heels to return to the starting position. That's one rep. Try to keep your back straight, chest up, and head looking straight ahead. Don't let the knees push out past the toes. Do the prescribed number of reps.

*If you have trouble with your knees going forward or you can't squat down far enough, try elevating your heels about an inch off the ground by standing on an inch-high board or weight plates and extend your arms straight out in front of you holding a light dumbbell.

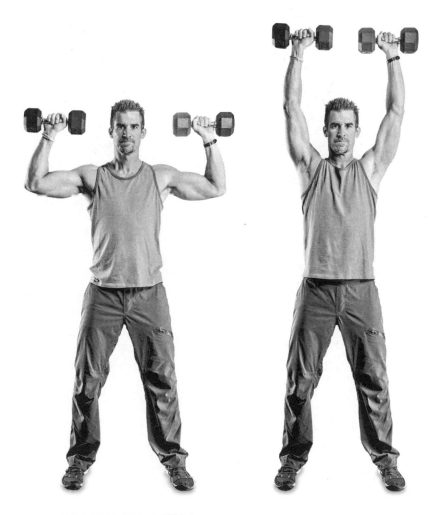

# STANDING MILITARY PRESS

Stand with your feet hip to shoulder-width apart and your knees slightly bent. Start with the dumbbells in front of your shoulders with your palms facing forward. Press the dumbbells straight above your head and bring the dumbbells together so that they almost touch when your arms are straight. Slowly lower the dumbbells back to the starting position at the shoulders. Repeat for the prescribed number of reps.

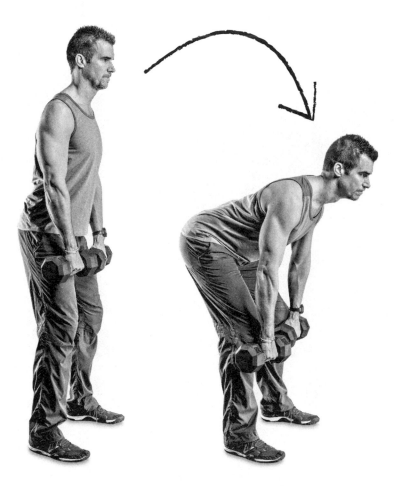

## ROMANIAN DEADLIFT (RDL)

Stand tall with your feet shoulder-width apart and your knees slightly bent. Hold a dumbbell in each hand in front of your thighs, palms facing in. Now, simultaneously push your butt back as you hinge forward at your hips, slowly lowering the dumbbells toward the ground. Keep the dumbbells close to your legs, your back flat, and your core muscles engaged throughout the movement. When you feel the stretch in your hamstrings (the weights do not have to touch the floor), slowly rise back up to the starting position by pushing your hips forward. That's one rep. Do the prescribed number of reps.

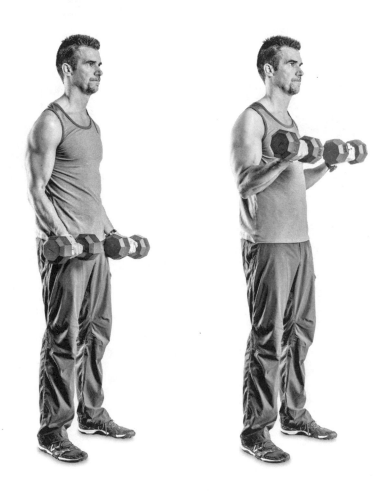

# BICEPS CURL

Stand holding a dumbbell in each hand with your arms in front of your thighs, palms facing up. Curl both dumbbells at the same time toward your shoulders in a controlled manner and then lower the dumbbells back to the starting position. That's one rep. Keep your elbows by your sides throughout the movement. Do the prescribed number of reps.

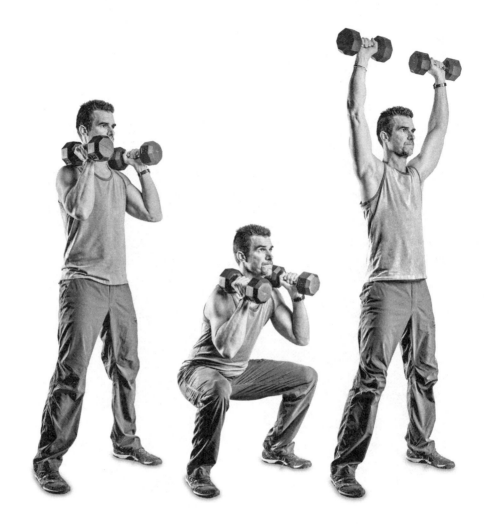

## SQUAT AND PRESS

Stand with your feet shoulder-width apart and hold a dumbbell in each hand in front of your shoulders with your palms facing in toward each other. Sit your butt back and bend your knees to squat until your thighs are parallel with the floor, then explosively press your heels into the floor as you straighten your legs. As you rise, use your momentum to help you press the dumbbells over your head in one continuous movement. Turn your palms forward as you reach the top position. Slowly bring the dumbbells back to your shoulders before performing the next rep. Do the prescribed number of reps.

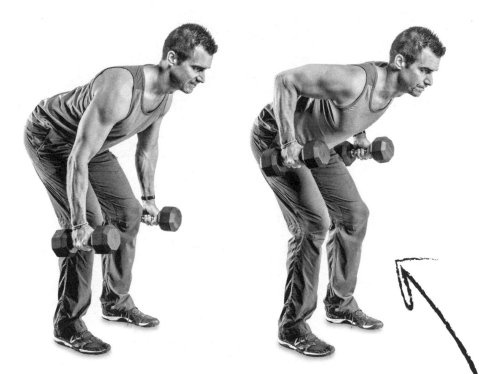

# ROW

With feet shoulder-width apart, grasp a dumbbell in each hand and lower yourself into the bottom of the RDL movement; that is, hinge forward at the hips and allow the dumbbells to lower toward the floor. When your back is nearly parallel with the floor, turn your wrists so your palms are facing each other. This is the starting position. Now, pull your elbows back using your back muscles so that the dumbbells come up close to your rib cage. Pause and then lower them back to the starting position. That's one rep. Do the prescribed number of reps.

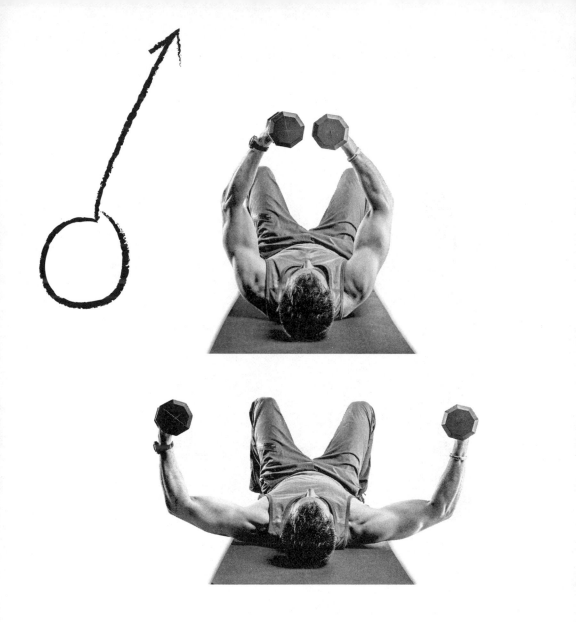

## CHEST FLY

Grasp two dumbbells and lie on your back on the floor (as shown) or on an exercise bench. Hold the weights above your chest with your elbows slightly bent and your palms facing each other. Keeping your elbows slightly bent, slowly lower the dumbbells out to your sides until you feel a stretch in your chest muscles. Next, bring the dumbbells back together in a hugging motion until the dumbbells nearly touch. That's one rep. Do the prescribed number of reps.

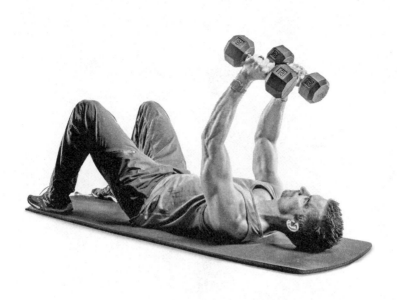

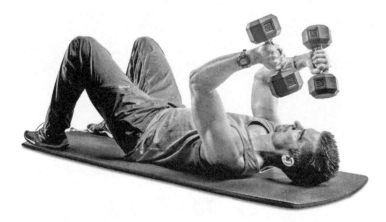

# TRICEPS EXTENSION

Lie on your back on the floor (as shown) or on an exercise bench, holding a dumbbell in each hand with arms extended over your chest. Your palms should face in toward each other. Now, slowly, lower the dumbbells toward your forehead without moving your upper arms, until your forearms are parallel with the floor. Pause and then slowly straighten your arms, pushing the dumbbells upward to the starting position. That's one rep. Do the prescribed number of reps.

# THE LEAN-OUT MEAL PLAN

## TRAIN HARD, EAT WELL

*In my best Arnold voice, ahem, "It's not a diet."*

**I DON'T LIKE THE WORD** *diet*. Why? Because as soon as you mention *diet* to someone, they get all cranky and start tossing out every excuse in the book as to why they weren't able to lose weight in the past. The word *diet* automatically conjures up images of teeny-tiny portions of kale salad, starvation, and failure.

Ask just about anyone and they'll tell you, "Diets don't work." In truth, diets don't fail; people do. Most people give up before they reach their goals, or they reach their goals and go back to eating fried chicken wings and waffles and ice cream and gain all their weight back, if not more. Plus, men don't diet! We eat, dammit! And eat we will. There's no "diet" per se in this book; instead, we call it the *Lean-Out Meal Plan*.

With this plan you'll learn the same eating strategies that I used to help Shaquille O'Neal shed 40 pounds in preparation for the TNT "shirt-off competition" against Charles Barkley. We're going to work hard and reward ourselves with good meals.

We're also going to keep this realistic. I'm not going to ask you to jump on some radical diet plan that will change who you are. I'm not going to ask you to go vegan if you're a meat-loving creature. I'm not going to suggest that you eat only organic foods or grapefruits or cabbage soup for 60 days straight. That would be nonsense.

Our 60-day plan emphasizes healthier food options that taste great; they're foods you'll want to eat. There's no starvation here—just better living. With all that said, if you want to lose weight and body fat, you have to burn off more calories than you consume. It's as simple as that!

### Calories In – More Calories Out = Weight Loss

With this plan, you can achieve weight loss and particularly fat loss in one of two ways:

1. You can train superhard, burn massive calories, and earn the ability to eat more calories per day, while dropping unwanted pounds and putting on some muscle.
2. You can phone in your exercise and consume fewer calories, way fewer!

It's your choice. Both will work.

Personally, I like option 1, so that's what I'm going to show you how to do. By burning more calories, you earn more food to eat. That way, you can eat more food and still lose weight. It's a win-win. See the calorie-calculating formulas on page 96.

# THE LEAN-OUT PLAN AT A GLANCE

The Lean-Out meal plan includes three meals and two snacks every day. The daily plan is detailed within each of the 4 quarters and Overtime period, beginning in Part III: Game Day. It's based on consuming 2,000 calories per day. Depending on how much you weigh and your activity level, you will likely need to adjust the daily plan to meet your specific calorie needs. I'll show you formulas to figure this out later on. This is a 60-day eating plan and each quarter and the OT period contains a helpful shopping list for exactly what you should purchase at the grocery story to get you through the 12 days. (You might have a lot of the stuff on the list already.) Some of the meals listed have specific recipes. You'll find these featured in Chapter 7. Look ahead a few days to see what you are going to be making, or to make meals ahead of time. This is a great way to keep committed to the plan. If you go thru the trouble of making the food you will be more likely to eat it—you won't fall off the wagon and eat junk food. Speaking of junk food, before starting this plan, go through your house and throw away the junk food. Plain and simple, just do it. If it's not in the house, then you won't be tempted to eat it. So throw it away, give it away, feed it to your dog, I don't care what you do with it—just get it out of the house. There is nothing radical in the Lean-Out plan; it's just eating sensible foods and controlling your portion size.

Now, you have another choice: You can start with the basic Lean-Out Plan in Quarter 1 or, if you're a gamer and want a head start on your competition, you'll begin with the 7-day Turbo Eating Plan detailed on page 103. It's a lot tougher than the basic Lean-Out, but a heck of a way to put on your game face. First, however, let's get some questions out of the way that I can tell are buzzing in your head:

## Q: Are you sure this isn't a diet?

*A:* Call it whatever you want to make you feel comfortable— a lifestyle change, an awakening, nutrition awareness, food counseling, a no-diet diet for dummies, "My Workout War Diet." I don't care; the words don't matter. Doing the work does!

## Q: Do I have to count calories?

*A:* I will answer your question with a question. Do you want to kick your friends' asses and win? Then yes, you'll count calories. A lot of weight-loss books promise "no calorie counting!" That's marketing baloney. If you don't monitor your calorie intake, how will you know if you are trimming enough to lose weight and body fat? Remember, you need to end the day with more calories gone than are added by the food you eat; that caloric deficit equates with getting leaner. If you decide not to count your calorie intake and expenditures, don't blame me if you lose your contest. I'm telling you to keep track of everything you do. It's only 60 days anyway, come on. Put pencil to paper or index finger to keyboard.

Are you a sports nut or a fantasy football guy? If so, think of it this way: It's like keeping the stats of your players. You're not going to start a running back or QB without checking out what he's been doing the past few weeks. It's the same with your eating. You have to keep your stats. Do it! Log your food. Check out "Sources, Templates, and Other Helpful Stuff" on page 256 for a food log you can copy along with apps and Web sites that make this quick and simple.

## Q: So what is the 60-day meal plan like?

*A:* As I mentioned earlier in the book, it's healthy eating, possibly much cleaner eating than you're doing now or have done in the past. It's 100 percent about giving your body the right amount of the right kind of fuel (food) in order to lose weight. Period. It's that simple. And it comes with a handy shopping list!

Ideally, I would like you to only eat clean, whole, unprocessed foods, but I know that isn't going to always happen. So instead of harping on you about it, I'm going to give you suggestions on what to eat, in case you have to eat out or eat something microwaved from a box or can.

# Q: How many meals do I get to eat?

**A:** You will eat no fewer than three meals per day plus two snacks.

# Q: How many calories will I need to eat every day?

**A:** Everyone's different. Your daily caloric amount will depend on your body's individual requirements. But the general meal plan provided is based on 2,000 calories per day broken down roughly like this:

Breakfast: 450 calories

Lunch: 500 calories

Snack: 250 calories

Dinner: 600 calories

Snack: 200 calories

As I mentioned earlier, for weight loss, you need to create a daily calorie deficit; that is, burn off more calories than you consume. If you're not using an online system or app to figure out how many calories you need to consume per day to lose weight, you'll need to do a little math. First calculate your basal metabolic rate, or BMR, which is the number of calories that you burn while at rest (in a 24-hour period). Basically, it's the number of calories it takes to run your body's machinery even if you are vegging out on the couch watching a game. Next, you have to estimate the number of calories you burn doing your typical daily activities. (If you work in an office, sitting at a desk all day, you'll burn fewer calories than someone who's doing manual labor in an 8- to 10-hour workday.) Adding those two numbers (BMR and activity calories) together gives you the number of calories your body requires to stay at your current weight. Take in more calories than that number and you'll gain weight. Get rid of more calories than you consume, and you'll lose weight.

Remember: 1 pound = 3,500 calories, so to lose 1 pound per week, you would need to restrict your daily intake by 500 calories per day, burn 500 calories per day, or accomplish some combination of both.

Below is the formula to calculate both numbers. If you don't want to mess with calculating and tracking things on your own, download a tracking app for your phone or computer. I highly recommend MyFitnessPal.com. Also, for a general guide to approximate calories in your favorite foods, see the sidebar on page 149.

## TO CALCULATE YOUR BASAL METABOLIC RATE (BMR):

» **Step 1.** Find your weight in kilograms (kg):
Your weight in pounds × .454 = your weight in kg

» **Step 2.** Find your height in centimeters (cm):
Your height in inches × 2.54 = your height in cm

» **Step 3.** Calculate: (10 × your weight in kg) + (6.25 × your height in cm) – (5 × your age in years) + 5 = BMR

## TO ESTIMATE YOUR ACTIVITY LEVEL:

» If you're sedentary (little or no exercise) = 1.2

» If you're lightly active (light exercise/sports 1–3 days/week) = 1.375

» If you're moderately active (moderate exercise/sports 3–5 days/week) = 1.55

» If you're very active (hard exercise/sports 6–7 days a week) = 1.725

» If you're extra active (very hard exercise/sports and physical job or twice-daily training) = 1.9

## TO CALCULATE YOUR DAILY ENERGY EXPENDITURE:

Your BMR × your activity level = total calories burned daily

## CALORIE DEFICIT NEEDED TO LOSE WEIGHT:

» 3,500 (calorie deficiency per week) or 500 per day to lose 1 pound per week

» 5,250 (calorie deficiency per week) or 750 per day to lose 1.5 pounds per week

» 7,000 (calorie deficiency per week) or 1,000 per day to lose 2 pounds per week

**EXAMPLE: BIG BELLY BILL**

Here's a typical guy: We'll call him Big Belly Bill. He's 70 inches tall, weighs 277.8 pounds, is 30 years old, and he works as an attorney for a fast-food company, so he knows from bacon double cheeseburgers. He would like to get his act together and lose about 1.5 pounds per week. So his formula looks like this:

**BMR = (10 × 126.12 kg) + (6.25 × 177.8 cm) − (5 × 30 yrs) + 5**

Bill's BMR = 2,227

Total calories burned = 2,227 × 1.2 (activity level)

Total calories burned to maintain current weight: 2,672

To lose weight: 2,672 − 750 (deficiency needed) = 1,922 (daily calorie goal)

## Q: Can I skip breakfast so I can eat more calories later in the day?

*A:* No way! Eating first thing in the morning keeps you from eating like a pig at a trough of slops later. Secondly, numerous research studies have suggested that people who eat breakfast tend to lose more weight and keep it off. A study by the National Weight Control Registry showed people who ate breakfast maintained a 30-pound (or more) weight loss for at least a year, and some as long as 6 years. Besides, aren't you hungry? You haven't eaten since last evening, maybe 10 or 12 hours ago. And besides, eggs and turkey or Canadian bacon taste pretty good at 7:00 a.m.!

## Q: What if I can't eat all five meals or reach my calorie goal?

*A:* Your food is your fuel for your workouts, your metabolism, and your daily life. Don't skip meals. Eat!

## Q: Do I have to buy everything on the shopping list?

*A:* No. Purchase only items that you don't already have, and you can substitute similar-calorie foods. For example, if my list says buy three bananas (and it does), but you don't like bananas, purchase some apples instead and adjust your calories accordingly. The lists are there for your convenience to help you plan ahead and avoid multiple trips to the store. They are more of an example than a prescription. Even the recipes in Chapter 7 are helpful suggestions, not requirements. I'm not here to force tilapia down your gullet.

## Q: What if I don't cook?

A: In the immortal words of my wife, Amy, "Suck it up, Gertrude!" Learn to cook. It's the single best way to control your nutrients and calories. Otherwise, you have to rely on someone else like that pimply-faced rising junior in the paper hat down at Bob's Burger-rama. You've got to eat, so if you don't have someone at home to help you, you're going to have to get creative. I know cooking can be a pain in the ass, especially when you are not prepared, meaning when you don't have the proper ingredients. I have put together a shopping list at the beginning of each quarter and overtime, along with that quarter's nutrition plan. This way you'll know what to eat and exactly what to buy, without guesswork.

If you absolutely have to eat most of your meals out, see "Dine Out and Still Win!" on page 149, and if you must toss something (frozen) in the microwave, I have a list of acceptable prepackaged items for you to choose from on page 108. When only a quickie will do, see the drinkable foods on page 146.

## Q: What do I do if I feel hungry?

A: Are you really hungry? Is your stomach growling? Or are you bored and wanting to eat out of habit? See "Rate Your Perceived Hunger," opposite. If you are experiencing true hunger:

- Make sure you are drinking enough water; this will help keep you feeling full and curb your appetite.
- Try to get in foods containing more fiber; this, too, will help with the feeling of fullness.

## Rate Your Perceived Hunger

We eat for a lot of reasons, and many of them have nothing to do with being hungry.

Think about it: How often have you scarfed half a bowl of chips just because it was sitting on the table in front of you? How many times have you gone up for seconds because everyone was going back to the buffet?

We eat when we're bored. Some of us eat when we're anxious or stressed. Often we confuse thirst with hunger and reach for a snack when what our bodies really want is a glass of water.

A big part of eating healthier (and consuming fewer calories) comes from developing into a more mindful eater. Before you go off half-cocked, shoveling food into your mouth by the fistful, stop long enough to ask yourself, "Am I really hungry?" On the chart here, you want to fly around 5. For best results, try not to ever get to a 2 or a 9.

| RATING | FEELING |
|:------:|:-------:|
| 1 | Famished |
| 2 | Extremely hungry |
| 3 | Hungry |
| 4 | First sign of hunger |
| 5 | Content |
| 6 | Somewhat full |
| 7 | Full |
| 8 | Very full |
| 9 | Stuffed |
| 10 | Beyond stuffed! |

- Suck it up! Seriously, this is a competition. You might be hungry once in a while, but show some stones and have some willpower.

## Q: Am I allowed to have a cocktail (or three)?

A: If you have the willpower, stay away from beer, wine, sangria, Long Island iced teas, fuzzy navels, and other alcoholic beverages. They are full of empty calories. All the effort you put into workouts will be wasted on adult beverages, so decline that craft beer and mix up a nice lime and sparkling water.

Think of it like this: You're in training camp, baby! And they're only taking the best guy: the guy who has what it takes to go all the way to the championship. If you want to be a baller, you've got to do the hard work. See how many days you can go without a drink. Optimally that would be all 60 days. I challenge you to see how many days you can go without popping a top or sipping on a cocktail.

# A LEG UP

## Keep Your Stats

Have you ever kept a scorecard when playing a round of golf? Or do you just go out there and hit the golf ball around, without counting strokes on each hole? I'm going to go out on a limb and guess your answer to that second question is "Hell, no!"

Like most golfers, you are meticulously counting on each hole and double-checking your score twice before going home. Heck, if you're like me, you also know exactly where your buddies stand on each hole.

We men love stats. We also collect and analyze data from our favorite teams, sports, and sports stars. If you've ever coached a recreational sports team, you know that keeping stats helps you change your lineup and game play, depending on which of your players are hitting the most free throws or batting in the most runs. So why should this be any different? You want your body to change, right? You want to crush your buddies into a bloody oblivion, right? Keep your stats!

Still need a little more coaxing? According to a study published by Kaiser Permanente's Center for Health Research, reported in the July 2008 issue of *Science Daily*, "Those who kept daily food records lost twice as much weight as those who kept no records." There's your proof!

It's said that the average person underestimates his or her *daily* food intake by 600 calories. That's more than a pound of body weight in excess calories per week! Keeping track of your calories in and calories out (through exercise) is the only way to make sure that you're hitting your goal. Think of your food journal as your own stats sheet; it's like a crystal ball that will reveal where your eating and exercise habits need adjustments. Without it, you're playing the game blind.

**Q: Should I take a multivitamin?**

*A:* Research on this is sketchy. Some experts say yes, while others say don't waste your money. I say err on the side of caution and take a multivitamin. As you ask more of your body physically, it needs more nutrients. Why not buy some safe insurance?

**Q: What if I make it through the first quarter, but the scale isn't moving. What's up? What can I do?**

*A:* The scale might not move in your favor every time you step onto it. Things that contribute to a not-so-great reading on the scale include:

## Getting Techy

While the thought of logging your calorie intake might seem like a tedious pain in the ass, here's a way to keep it simple. Go onto MyFitnessPal.com and sign up for a free account. This is the same system we used to track Shaq's calories, and it's how readers of my wife's book, *Six Weeks to Skinny Jeans*, track theirs. Why do we all use it? Because it's extremely quick and user-friendly, and you can gauge where you are with a quick glance at your home page. They even have a cool app for your phone.

After you scan a food bar code, the app will automatically search the database for your item and log it into your journal for you. With this free tool, you can log your food and exercise wherever and whenever you'd like, even if you can't get to a computer.

At the time of publication, there are mobile apps for iPhone, iPod, Android, BlackBerry, and Windows Phone 7. Your MyFitnessPal account is always at your fingertips. These apps work with the Web site, giving you access to the same comprehensive database of more than 2,222,000 foods and restaurant items. Any changes you make on your phone will be synchronized to the Web and vice versa, so you always have complete and up-to-date access to your account.

On this same site, you can also keep track of your buddies and trash talk them, right there on your page. And you can join our Workout War community board on MyFitnessPal. While you're there, friend me—my user name is JimCotta.

If you're not one of those guys who love technology and you like putting ink to paper, you can still log your eating and exercise by using the template on page 257. Just make copies of it and keep it with you at *all* times.

So what are you waiting for? Put the book down and go do this, now!

- The time of day you weigh yourself. If you weigh yourself right after eating or drinking a bunch of water or other liquids, you're gonna weigh slightly more.

- How much undigested food you still have in your stomach and intestines. You've heard the term "full of shit." Well, you just might be.

- You might be putting on lean muscle, in which case, your clothes will be fitting a little less snug, but the scale isn't budging. This means your body composition is changing for the better! And no, muscle doesn't weigh more than fat; it's just a lot better to have hanging on your skeleton.

- Weigh yourself only once per week. If you have to do it daily, do it first thing in the morning, after going to the bathroom and before getting dressed. This will give you the most accurate weight for the day. And know that no two scales will weigh you the same, so use the same scale each time.
- Give yourself a checkup . . .
  - *Are you eating every 2 to 3 hours? You should be!*
  - *Are you counting the calories you drink? You should be!*
  - *Are you working out as the plan is prescribed? If no, then start. If yes, you might be putting on lean muscle, in which case your body composition is changing and the scale won't always reflect your true changes.*
  - *Go back and recalculate your calories.*
  - *For a few days, reduce your calories by 150 per day, making sure to never go below 1,500.*

## Q: How is the Turbo Eating Plan different from the Lean-Out Plan?

*A:* It's hardcore. It's much like what bodybuilders do to rip up right before a competition. It's by no means a lifestyle way of eating, but when used properly, it quickly gets the job done. It's for the guy who isn't joking around; it's a 7-day kick in the pants to put you on the right track! I'll show you how to get it done on the next page.

Enough with the chitchat, ladies. Let's get started.

# THE TURBO EATING PLAN

This is a 7-day program for accelerated weight loss, and it isn't for the faint of heart. If you're not joking around and you're okay with kicking your own ass in order to kick the competition's, this plan is for you.

In order to crush the competition, you're going to eat low- to moderate-GI (glycemic index) foods and lean protein sources for the first 7 days. Then on day 8, you'll jump into the normal Lean-Out eating plan. This jump-start will help lean you out and trim pounds like crazy.

So what are you looking at for 7 days?

- Zero fruit or sugar of any kind
- Zero alcohol
- Zero bread or pasta products
- Only clean, low-GI foods and lean protein sources
- No calorie counting

If you're ready to kick it into high gear, check out the Turbo Eating Plan Cheat Sheet on page 104. It contains everything you can eat and some items that are strictly forbidden. Unlike the Lean-Out Meal Plan, you are *not* counting calories here. You'll eat until you feel content and not stuffed. You'll eat three meals and two snacks. You're trying to maintain a constant state of happiness, meaning you should never feel like you're starving. Make sure you are drinking, at a minimum, 64 ounces of water per day.

## Turbo Eating Plan Survival Tips

1. Make your food in advance and in bulk. Set aside some time and pre-package snacks in individual resealable plastic bags or containers. If you have enough, make them for the entire week. When making dinner, prepare enough that you can also have it for lunch the next day. If you are making a soup, stew, or some sort of casserole, double up the recipe and eat it for several meals. Keep plenty of approved snacks handy at home, in your car, and at work.
2. Don't be stingy with the flavoring of your food. Let's face it: If what you're eating isn't tasty, you're most likely not going to want to eat it, and you might find yourself eating something that's not on the plan.
3. Drink lots and lots and lots of water. This will keep you feeling full.

# Turbo Eating Plan Cheat Sheet

| YES! | | NO! | |
|------|------|------|------|

## BEANS/LEGUMES

| | | | |
|------|------|------|------|
| Adzuki beans | Kidney beans | | |
| Black beans | Lentils | | |
| Black-eyed peas | Lima beans | | |
| Broad beans | Navy beans | | |
| Butter beans | Pigeon peas | | |
| Cannellini beans | Pinto beans | | |
| Chickpeas or garbanzo beans | Soybeans | | |
| | Split peas | | |
| Great Northern beans | White beans | | |
| Italian beans | | | |

*Enjoy the Yes! items; avoid those listed as No!*

## CHEESE

| | | | |
|------|------|------|------|
| Laughing Cow light cheese | Lower-fat ricotta | All full-fat cheese or cream cheese | |
| Lower-fat cottage cheese | Parmesan | | |
| | Part-skim mozzarella | | |
| Lower-fat cream cheese | Reduced-fat Cheddar or feta | | |

## EGGS AND OTHER DAIRY PRODUCTS

| | | | |
|------|------|------|------|
| Eggs | Lower-fat sour cream | Chocolate milk | Queso dip |
| Fat-free milk | | Full-fat milk | Watch out for soymilks (most have high sugar content) |
| I Can't Believe It's Not Butter! | Smart Balance olive oil spread | Full-fat sour cream | |
| Liquid egg whites | Sugar-free yogurt | Ice cream | |
| Lower-fat plain or Greek yogurt | | | |

| YES! | | NO! | |
|---|---|---|---|
| **FATS/OILS** | | | |
| Canola | Peanut | Butter | Palm |
| Corn | Sesame | Lard and other | Vegetable |
| Enova | Soybean | solid shortening | |
| Flaxseed | Sunflower | | |
| Grapeseed | Walnut | | |
| Extra-virgin olive oil | | | |
| **FRUIT** | | | |
| Lemons and limes | | All other fruits and fruit juices | |
| **BEEF AND PORK** | | | |
| Bison | Lean ground sirloin | Fatty cuts of beef (brisket, liver, etc.) | Ham with honey or maple |
| Canadian bacon | | | |
| Lean beef tenderloin | Lean sirloin steaks | | |
| | Tri tip steaks | | |
| **VEGETABLES** | | | |
| Artichokes | Green bell peppers | Beets | White/sweet potatoes |
| Asparagus | | Carrots | |
| Avocado | Lettuce (all types) | Corn | Yams |
| Bell peppers | Mixed greens | | |
| Broccoli | Mushrooms | | |
| Cabbage | Onions | | |
| Cauliflower | Snow peas | | |
| Celery | Spinach | | |
| Collard greens | Squash | | |
| Cucumbers | Tomatoes | | |
| Eggplant | Zucchini | | |
| Green beans | | | |

| YES! | | NO! | |
|------|------|------|------|
| **POULTRY** | | | |
| Chicken breast | Turkey bacon | Chicken wings or legs | Processed poultry (nuggets or fingers) |
| Deli turkey or chicken | White-meat turkey | Duck | |
| Ground turkey | | Goose | |
| **SEAFOOD** | | | |
| Canned crabmeat | Swordfish | Breaded and fried fish | |
| Halibut | Tilapia | | |
| Mahimahi | Tuna steak | | |
| Salmon | Water-packed canned tuna | | |
| Scallops | | | |
| Shrimp | | | |
| Sole | | | |
| **SOY, NUTS, BEANS** | | | |
| Almonds (dry roasted) | Pistachios | Cashews | |
| Black beans | Red kidney beans | Macadamia nuts | |
| Chickpeas | Tempeh | | |
| Edamame | Tofu | | |
| Hummus | Walnuts | | |
| Pine nuts | White beans | | |
| Pinto beans | | | |
| **DRINKS** | | | |
| Coffee (black or with fat-free milk) | Regular or sparkling water | Alcohol (beer, wine, liquor) | Fruit juice |
| Green, black, or herbal tea | V8 tomato juice | Energy drinks | Regular soda |
| | | | Sugary coffee drinks |
| **SNACKS** | | | |
| Sugar-free ice pops | Sugar-free pudding and Jell-O | All cookies | Doughnuts |
| | | Cakes | Pies |
| | | Candy bars | |

# THE LEAN-OUT RECIPES

## DELICIOUS BODY-CHANGING MEALS FOR WARRIORS

**IF YOU PLAN ON SPANKING YOUR COMPETITION AND WALKING AWAY WITH THE PRIZE, COOKING YOUR MEALS IS ESSENTIAL.** You can't live on takeout, cold cuts, and frozen dinners and expect to have washboard abs. A regular diet of restaurant food and premade packaged meals will give you a gut ... guaranteed.

The proven way to fast weight loss is by making your own breakfasts, lunches, dinners, and snacks. Cooking gives you control over ingredients, calories, sodium content, and portion size. When you prepare your meals, you manage the quality of the fuel that goes into your body. There is no greater way to positively influence your health immediately.

In this chapter, you'll find easy and delicious recipes for many of the meals in the quarter-by-quarter 60-day plans starting on page 167.

## Healthy Packaged Foods Cheat Sheet

I know there will be times when you just don't have time to make home-made lentil soup or roast a turkey or even grill a steak. You have to eat on the fly. That's when it's handy to have some frozen and prepackaged foods nearby that you can count on to be relatively healthful (i.e., low in sodium, calories, and preservatives). Here are some of my favorites to consider.

### Breakfast

Bagel-fuls
Kashi 7-Grain Waffles
Dannon Light & Fit Greek Yogurt
Smart Ones Smart Beginnings
breakfast sandwiches
Special K Flatbread breakfast sandwich

### Lunch and Dinner

Bagel Bites
Healthy Choice 100% Natural Café Steamers
Healthy Choice Top Chef Café Steamers
Hormel REV Wraps

Kashi Thin Crust Mediterranean Pizza
Lean Cuisine frozen entrees
Lean Pockets sandwiches

### Snack and Deserts

Healthy Choice Greek Frozen Yogurt
Jell-O Sugar Free Pudding in
reduced-fat or fat-free varieties
Orville Redenbacher's Gourmet Naturals
Simply Salted Popcorn
Skinny Cow frozen treats
and/or candy varieties

# BREAKFASTS

## BREAKFAST BURRITO

3    egg whites

1    cup Birds Eye Recipe Ready Chopped Green Peppers
     and Onions

1    flour tortilla (6"), such as Mission Carb Balance

2    tablespoons tomato salsa

3    tablespoons reduced-fat shredded cheese

**MAKE IT**

Scramble the egg whites, adding in the vegetable mixture.

Spread the mixture over the tortilla. (You can warm the tortilla quickly in the microwave for 3 to 5 seconds, if desired.) Top with the salsa and cheese.

Roll up tightly into a wrap. Eat right away or wrap tightly in plastic wrap for another day.

*Makes 1 serving*

**Per serving:** 354 calories, 33 g protein, 12 g fat, 31 g carbohydrates

# BAKED BREAKFAST PEPPERS

| | |
|---|---|
| 2 | large red bell peppers |
| 4 | strips turkey bacon |
| 4 | egg whites |
| 1 | tablespoon milk |
| | Dash of salt |
| ¼ | teaspoon black pepper |
| ¼ | cup low-fat shredded Cheddar cheese, divided |
| ¼ | teaspoon garlic powder |

**MAKE IT**

Preheat the oven to 375°F.

Wash and cut the peppers in half lengthwise, removing the seeds. Make sure to leave the stems intact.

Lightly coat a baking sheet with nonstick cooking spray. Place the peppers on the sheet so they resemble cups. Place in the oven and bake until soft, about 9 to 10 minutes.

While the peppers are cooking, cook the bacon. Let it cool and then break it up into pieces.

In a small bowl, whisk the egg whites, milk, salt, pepper, and half of the cheese.

Place the egg mixture into the pepper cups along with the crunched-up bacon.

Place the peppers back in the oven and bake until the eggs set and look puffy in the center, about 20 to 25 minutes.

Garnish with the remaining cheese and garlic powder.

**Note:** You can also top with cilantro, avocado, or salsa, making sure to add in the calories for any additions. You can double or triple this recipe and keep the remaining portions in airtight containers to eat tomorrow and the following day, warming them up in the microwave.

*Makes 4 servings*

**Per serving (1 pepper cup):** 210 calories, 18 g protein, 11 g fat, 3 g carbohydrates

# FRENCH TOAST

1    slightly beaten egg

1    slightly beaten egg white

¾    cup fat-free milk

⅛    teaspoon ground cinnamon

1½   teaspoons vanilla extract

8    slices French bread, ½" thick

**MAKE IT**

Preheat the oven to 450°F.

Coat a large baking sheet with nonstick cooking spray.

Mix together the egg, egg white, milk, cinnamon, and vanilla.

Dip the bread slices into the egg mixture just long enough to coat both sides.

Place on the baking sheet and bake until the bread is lightly brown, about 6 minutes.

Turn the bread over and bake for another 5 to 8 minutes.

Optional: Top with sugar-free syrup (not included in calories).

*Makes 4 servings*

**Per serving (2 slices):** 245 calories, 13 g protein, 2 g fat, 50 g carbohydrates

## TUNA PITA SANDWICH

| | |
|---|---|
| 1 | can (6.5 ounces) tuna (water packed) |
| ¼ | cup finely chopped dill pickle |
| ¼ | cup finely chopped celery (optional) |
| 2 | tablespoons reduced-fat olive oil mayonnaise |
| 1½ | teaspoons prepared mustard |
| 3 | lettuce leaves |
| 3 | small whole wheat pita pockets, top cut |

**MAKE IT**

Strain and rinse the tuna.

Place the tuna in a small bowl and break it up with a fork.

Add the pickle, celery, mayonnaise, and mustard. Mix together.

Divide the mixture up into 3 servings. Place 2 of the servings in an airtight container for lunch the next 2 days. Set 2 lettuce leaves and 2 pitas aside as well.

Place the remaining mixture in the remaining pita half along with the remaining lettuce and enjoy.

*Makes 3 servings*

**Per serving (1 sandwich):** 139 calories, 10 g protein, 3 g fat, 18 g carbohydrates

# CHICKEN CURRY SALAD

1½   teaspoons Dijon mustard

1     tablespoon reduced-fat olive oil mayonnaise

1     teaspoon sugar or 1 Splenda packet

½     cup plain fat-free Greek yogurt

½     teaspoon curry powder

⅓     cup diagonally sliced celery

⅛     teaspoon salt

2     cups diced, cooked chicken breast

2     teaspoons lemon juice

⅔     cup diced, unpeeled Red Delicious apple

      Dash of black pepper

**MAKE IT**

Mix all ingredients together in a large bowl.

*Makes 3 servings*

**Per serving:** 234 calories, 33 g protein, 4 g fat, 13 g carbohydrates

# MEATBALL SANDWICH

2   cups pasta sauce

12  frozen cooked meatballs

4   whole wheat hot dog buns

1½  cups shredded mozzarella cheese or grated Parmesan
    cheese, divided

**MAKE IT**

In a small saucepan, heat the sauce over medium. Place the meatballs into the
sauce and bring to a boil. Reduce the heat to low, stirring occasionally. Cover
and cook until the meatballs are heated through, about 20 minutes.

Portion the meatballs out into 4 servings. Place the unused servings into an
airtight container for a meal at a later date.

Put the meatballs for your sandwich on a roll and sprinkle with one-quarter of
the cheese. The remaining cheese is for the remaining sandwiches.

*Makes 4 servings*

**Per serving (1 sandwich):** 274 calories, 15 g protein, 2 g fat, 16 g carbohydrates

# TACO SALAD

1    cup black beans or Black Bean Dip (page 143)

10   baked blue corn tortilla chips

3    cups salad greens (shredded lettuce or chopped romaine is great)

1    cup broccoli slaw (shredded raw mix in bag)

1    cup onion and bell pepper, sliced and sautéed using nonstick cooking spray

¼    cup reduced-fat shredded cheese

½    cup tomato salsa

2    tablespoons guacamole

**MAKE IT**

Drain and rinse the black beans (or use Black Bean Dip).

Place the chips on a plate or in a large bowl. Top the chips with the salad greens and broccoli slaw. Place the sautéed onion and pepper on top of the greens. Spread the beans or dip over the mixture in the plate or bowl. Sprinkle with the cheese and top with the salsa and guacamole.

*Makes 1 serving*

**Per serving:** 577 calories, 28 g protein, 18 g fat, 85 g carbohydrates

# FRUIT AND ALMOND SALAD

| | |
|---|---|
| 1 | teaspoon honey |
| ½ | teaspoon Dijon mustard |
| ¼ | cup vanilla fat-free Greek yogurt |
| 1 | Gala apple, sliced |
| 1 | green apple, sliced |
| ½ | cup fresh blueberries |
| ¼ | cup toasted sliced almonds |
| 3 | cups spinach |

**MAKE IT**

In a small bowl, combine the honey, mustard, and yogurt. Mix well.

In a large bowl, combine the apples, blueberries, almonds, and spinach.

Toss the dressing with the ingredients in the large bowl.

*Makes 2 servings*

**Per serving:** 220 calories, 8 g protein, 7 g fat, 37 g carbohydrates

# DINNERS

## GRILLED TILAPIA FILLETS

| 4 | tilapia fillets (4 ounces each) |
| 4 | teaspoons extra-virgin olive oil |
| ½ | cup orange juice |
| 4 | slices onion |

**MAKE IT**

Wrap each fillet in aluminum foil, but leave the top open to put in other ingredients. Cover each piece of tilapia with 1 teaspoon olive oil, 2 tablespoons orange juice, and 1 onion slice. Now cover up the tilapia with the foil so it's sealed tight.

Heat a grill to high heat. Place the foil-wrapped fish on the grill and cook for 6 minutes. Carefully remove the fish from the foil and place on a plate.

*Makes 4 servings*

**Per serving (1 fillet):** 187 calories, 29 g protein, 7 g fat, 2 g carbohydrates

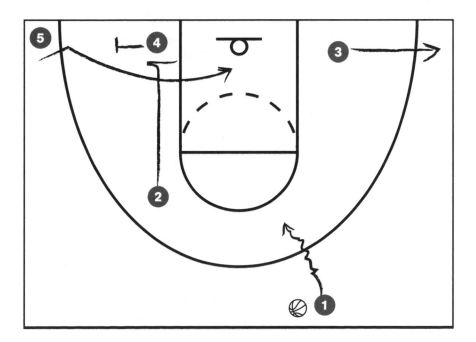

# FIX AND FORGET ENCHILADA SOUP

| | |
|---|---|
| 1 | can (15 ounces) black beans, rinsed and drained |
| 1 | can (14.5 ounces) diced tomatoes |
| 1 | chopped onion |
| 1 | can (15 ounces) whole kernel corn or 10 ounces frozen |
| 1 | bunch fresh cilantro |
| 1 | tablespoon crushed red pepper |
| 1 | can Campbell's 98% Fat-Free Cream of Chicken soup |
| 1½ | cups fat-free milk |
| 1 | packet taco seasoning |
| 1 | pound chicken tenderloins or chicken breasts |

**MAKE IT**

Place the beans, tomatoes, onion, corn, cilantro, and crushed pepper in a slow cooker and stir together.

In a small bowl, mix together the soup, milk, and taco seasoning. Set aside.

Place the chicken breast in the slow cooker on top of the bean mixture. Pour the soup mixture over the chicken. Cover and cook on low for 6 to 8 hours.

Before serving, remove the chicken and shred it. Add the chicken back to the soup.

**Note:** You can serve the soup with low-fat sour cream and cheese, making sure to account for the added calories. Nutrition information is for the soup only.

*Makes 12 servings*

**Per serving:** 143 calories, 12 g protein, 2 g fat, 18 g carbohydrates

# GRILLED PORK CHOPS

4    boneless pork chops (center-cut loin, 4 ounces each)
1    teaspoon salt
1    teaspoon black pepper
½    cup salsa verde

**MAKE IT**

Heat the grill to high heat. Season the pork chops with salt and pepper.

Grill the pork chops for 3 minutes per side. Top each chop with 2 tablespoons salsa verde.

*Makes 4 servings*

**Per serving (1 chop):** 180 calories, 32 g protein, 6 g fat, 0 g carbohydrates


# SALMON CAKES

1    egg white
1    teaspoon lemon juice
¼    cup chopped green onion
¼    cup seasoned bread crumbs
1    can (18 ounces) boneless salmon or crabmeat, drained
     Black pepper and garlic powder to taste

**MAKE IT**

In a large bowl, combine all ingredients. Divide into 8 portions (about ⅓ cup each) and make each portion into a patty.

Coat a skillet with cooking spray and cook over medium-high heat, about 4 minutes for each side of the cakes.

*Makes 8 cakes*

**Per serving (2 cakes):** 171 calories, 25 g protein, 5 g fat, 6 g carbohydrates

# CHICKEN FAJITAS

| | |
|---|---|
| 8 | flour tortillas (6"), such as Mission Carb Balance |
| 1 | small onion, sliced and separated into rings |
| 2 | cloves garlic, minced |
| 1 | medium red or green bell pepper, cut into bite-size strips |
| 1 | tablespoon extra-virgin olive oil |
| 8 | ounces boned skinless chicken breast halves, cut into bite-size strips |
| ⅓ | cup tomato salsa |
| 2 | cups shredded lettuce |
| ¼ | cup plain low-fat yogurt or low-fat sour cream |

**MAKE IT**

Preheat the oven to 300°F. Wrap the tortillas in foil and place in the oven for 10 to 12 minutes.

Coat a skillet with nonstick cooking spray. Cook the onion and garlic for about 2 minutes. Add the bell pepper and cook until tender, about 2 minutes. Remove the vegetables from the skillet and set aside.

Add the oil to the pan. Add the chicken and cook for 3 to 5 minutes, or until it is no longer pink. Add the vegetables to the skillet and add the salsa. Cook until the mixture is heated through.

Divide the chicken into fourths, adding chicken on top of each tortilla.

Top each tortilla with shredded lettuce, and yogurt.

*Makes 4 servings*

**Per serving (2 fajitas):** 319 calories, 28 g protein, 8 g fat, 36 g carbohydrates

# MA... THE MEAT LOAF

1    pound ground turkey
1    box whole wheat stuffing mix
1    cup water
2    whole eggs
4    tablespoons ketchup, divided

**MAKE IT**

Preheat the oven to 400°F.

In a medium mixing bowl, stir together the turkey, stuffing mix, water, eggs, and 1 tablespoon of the ketchup.

Place the mixture in a loaf pan and bake for about 40 to 45 minutes. Pull the meat loaf out of the oven and top with the remaining ketchup.

Place the loaf back into the oven and bake for another 10 minutes, or until done.

*Makes 8 servings*

**Per serving:** 129 calories, 13 g protein, 2 g fat, 15 g carbohydrates

*Just like your mama makes*

# FISH AND CHIPS SALAD

2    tablespoons extra-virgin olive oil, divided

4    small Yukon Gold potatoes, cut into thin round slices

Pinch of salt

1    medium shallot, thinly sliced

2    teaspoons rice vinegar

¼    cup low-fat buttermilk

2    cans (7 ounces each) boneless, skinless salmon, drained

8    cups arugula

## MAKE IT

Heat 1 tablespoon of the oil in a large skillet over medium-high heat.

Add the potato slices and cook, turning halfway through cooking (5 minutes per side). Transfer to a plate and sprinkle lightly with salt.

Combine the shallot, the remaining 1 tablespoon oil, and the vinegar in a small saucepan. Bring to a boil over medium heat. Remove from the heat and whisk in the buttermilk.

Place the salmon in a medium bowl, add the warm dressing, and toss. Place the salmon mixture on top of the potatoes. Top with arugula to serve.

*Makes 4 servings*

**Per serving:** 260 calories, 24 g protein, 10 g fat, 15 g carbohydrates

# EASY PULLED PORK

2     pounds pork tenderloin, trimmed

1     cup diet root beer

1¼   cups barbecue sauce

**MAKE IT**

Set a slow cooker to low. Rinse off the tenderloin and pat it dry. Brown the tenderloin (on all sides) in a nonstick skillet. Place the tenderloin in the slow cooker. Pour the root beer into the cooker and cover the top of the tenderloin with barbecue sauce.

Cook on low until you can easily pull the pork apart with a fork, approximately 4 to 6 hours.

*Makes 8 servings*

**Per serving:** 276 calories, 35 g protein, 9 g fat, 11 g carbohydrates

# GRILLED JERK CHICKEN

4     boneless, skinless chicken breasts (6 ounces each)

2     teaspoons jerk seasoning

**MAKE IT**

Season the chicken with ½ teaspoon jerk seasoning per breast.

Heat a grill to high heat. Cook on the grill for 7 to 8 minutes per side.

*Makes 4 servings*

**Per serving:** 180 calories, 39 g protein, 2 g fat, 0 g carbohydrates

# FISH AND BEAN TOSTADAS

8    small (6") corn tortillas

1    can (6–7 ounces) boneless, skinless wild Alaskan salmon, drained

1    avocado, diced

2    tablespoons minced pickled jalapeños, plus 2 tablespoons pickling juice from the jar, divided

2    cups coleslaw mix or shredded cabbage

2    tablespoons chopped fresh cilantro

1    can (15 ounces) black beans, rinsed

2    scallions, chopped

2    tablespoons tomato salsa

3    tablespoons reduced-fat sour cream

    Lime wedges (optional)

### MAKE IT

Preheat the oven to 375°F. Spray each side of the tortillas with nonstick cooking spray.

Place the tortillas on baking sheets. Bake, turning once, until light brown, 12 to 14 minutes.

Combine the salmon, avocado, and jalapeños in a bowl. Combine the cabbage, cilantro, and the pickling juice in another bowl.

Process the black beans, scallions, salsa, and sour cream in a food processor until smooth (or just smash well with fork). Transfer to a microwave-safe bowl.

Cover and microwave on high until hot, about 2 minutes.

To assemble the tostadas, spread each tortilla with bean mixture and salmon mixture and top with the cabbage salad.

Serve with lime wedges, if desired.

*Makes 4 servings*

**Per serving (2 tostadas):** 319 calories, 16 g protein, 11 g fat, 43 g carbohydrates

# CRAB-BAKED AVOCADOS

| | |
|---|---|
| 4 | large ripe avocados |
| 1 | can crabmeat |
| 1 | can medium shrimp |
| 1 | cup reduced-fat olive oil mayonnaise |
| 1 | tablespoon lemon juice |
| ½ | cup finely chopped onion |
| ⅛ | teaspoon salt |
| ⅛ | teaspoon black pepper |

**MAKE IT**

Preheat the oven to 350°F. Cut the avocados in half and remove the pits.

Drain the crabmeat, flake it with a fork, and remove any cartilage. Drain and rinse the shrimp. In a bowl, mix together the mayonnaise, lemon juice, onion, salt, and pepper.

Add the crab and shrimp to the mixture.

Place the mixture into the avocado halves.

Place the avocado halves into an ungreased 13" x 9" baking dish.

Baked uncovered until the mixture is bubbly, about 25 to 30 minutes.

*Makes 4 servings*

**Per serving (2 avocado halves):** 472 calories, 15 g protein, 38 g fat, 16 g carbohydrates

# BLACK BEANS AND RICE

1    large onion

2    cans (15 ounces each) fat-free black beans

3¾   cups reduced-sodium chicken broth

1½   cups uncooked brown rice

2    teaspoons ground cumin

1    teaspoon salt

3    cloves garlic

1    tablespoon lime juice

**MAKE IT**

Chop the onion and rinse the beans.

Place all the ingredients except the beans into a slow cooker and mix well.

Cover and allow to cook for about 7½ hours on low. The rice will be tender.

Stir in the beans and allow to cook for another 15 to 20 minutes.

Top with light sour cream if you wish.

*Makes 6 servings*

**Per serving:** 241 calories, 14 g protein, 1 g fat, 43 g carbohydrates

# EASY BEEF STEW

2   medium green bell peppers

2   medium yellow onions

1   tablespoon seasoning salt

1   teaspoon black pepper

2   cans (14 ounces each) diced tomatoes, undrained

4   pounds boneless beef tips

## MAKE IT

Cut the bell peppers into ½" strips and dice the onions. Place all the ingredients into a slow cooker. Mix the ingredients well and cover. Set the cooker on low and cook for about 8 hours. The meat should be tender.

*Makes 10 servings*

**Per serving:** 227 calories, 21 g protein, 12 g fat, 8 g carbohydrates

*Even you can make this one!*

# ASIAN PEANUT NOODLES

1   pound boneless, skinless chicken breasts

2   tablespoons reduced-sodium soy sauce

2   tablespoons minced garlic

1   teaspoon minced fresh ginger

½   cup smooth peanut butter

1½  teaspoons chili-garlic sauce, or to taste

8   ounces whole wheat spaghetti

1   bag (12 ounces) frozen vegetable medley, such as carrots, broccoli, and snow peas

**MAKE IT**

Put a large pot of water on to boil for cooking the pasta.

Place the chicken in a skillet or saucepan, add enough water to cover, and bring to a boil.

Cover, reduce the heat to low, and simmer gently until cooked through and no longer pink in the middle, 10 to 12 minutes. Transfer the chicken to a cutting board. When it's cool enough to handle, shred it into bite-size strips.

Whisk the soy sauce, garlic, ginger, peanut butter, and chili-garlic sauce in a large bowl. Cook the pasta in the boiling water until not quite tender, about 1 minute less than specified in the package directions. Add the vegetables and cook until the pasta and vegetables are just tender, 1 minute more. Drain, reserving 1 cup of the cooking liquid.

Rinse the pasta and vegetables with cool water to refresh and stop the cooking process. Stir the reserved cooking liquid into the peanut sauce. Add the pasta, vegetables, and chicken; toss well to coat.

*Makes 6 servings*

**Per serving (1½ cups):** 363 calories, 29 g protein, 12 g fat, 36 g carbohydrates

# SPICY VEGETARIAN CHILI

2   bags Birds Eye Recipe Ready Southwest Blend

1   tablespoon extra-virgin olive oil

1   can (14.5 ounces) diced tomatoes

4   cups water, or for added flavor, use vegetable stock

3   tablespoons tomato paste

1   can (4 ounces) chopped green chiles

½   cup chili powder

2   tablespoons salt

1   tablespoon cumin

**MAKE IT**

In a deep saucepan over medium-high heat, sauté the frozen vegetable mix and oil for about 3 minutes. Add the tomatoes, water or stock, tomato paste, and chiles. Bring to a boil, stirring often.

Turn the heat down to a simmer and add the chili powder, salt, and cumin. Cook for another 20 to 25 minutes. If you like, you can garnish with cilantro.

*Makes 4 servings*

**Per serving:** 63 calories, 3 g protein, 1 g fat, 12 g carbohydrates

For meatless Mondays!

# SHRIMP AND EDAMAME

| | |
|---|---|
| 2 | slices turkey bacon |
| 1 | tablespoon extra-virgin olive oil |
| 1 | bunch scallions or 1 small onion, sliced |
| 1 | red bell pepper, diced |
| 1½ | teaspoons fresh thyme or 1 teaspoon dried |
| 2 | cloves garlic, minced |
| 1 | tablespoon cider vinegar |
| 1 | package (10 ounces) frozen shelled edamame |
| ½ | cup reduced-sodium chicken or vegetable broth |
| 1 | package (10 ounces) frozen corn |
| | Pinch of salt |
| 1 | bag (1 pound, 26–30 count) frozen cooked/peeled/cleaned shrimp |

## MAKE IT

Cook the bacon in a skillet. Keep the bacon drippings in the pan and move the bacon to paper towels to cool.

Add the oil to the pan along with the scallions or onion, bell pepper, thyme, and garlic. Stir and cook for 3 minutes. Add the vinegar, edamame, broth, corn, and salt.

Bring to a simmer and reduce the heat to medium-low. Cook for 5 minutes.

Add the shrimp on top of the veggies, cover the pot, and cook for 5 minutes more. Remove from the heat and crumble the bacon on top.

*Makes 4 servings*

**Per serving:** 307 calories, 30 g protein, 9 g fat, 26 g carbohydrates

# GREEK ORZO SALAD

| | |
|---|---|
| 1 | tablespoon extra-virgin olive oil |
| ½ | cup crumbled feta cheese |
| ½ | cup kalamata olives, pitted |
| 2 | cups whole wheat orzo, cooked |
| 2 | Roma tomatoes, sliced |
| 3 | cups fresh baby spinach |

**MAKE IT**

Toss the above ingredients together. (You can save a portion for later in the day; toss again with fresh spinach leaves.)

*Makes 2 servings*

**Per serving:** 446 calories, 13 g protein, 21 g fat, 52 g carbohydrates

*Makes a great lunch, too!*

# GRILLED SWEET POTATOES

| | |
|---|---|
| 2 | pounds sweet potatoes |
| 1 | teaspoon lemon or lime zest |
| 3 | tablespoons extra-virgin olive oil |
| 2 | teaspoons fresh lime or lemon juice |
| ¼ | cup finely chopped fresh cilantro |
| | Pinch of salt |

**MAKE IT**

Prepare a grill for direct, hot heat.

Puncture the potatoes with a knife or fork and place in the microwave for 2 minutes to soften them to cut. Peel the potatoes and slice them lengthwise into ¼"-thick pieces.

In a bowl, combine the lemon or lime zest, olive oil, lime or lemon juice, and cilantro.

Place the potato slices in the bowl, coat the potatoes with the lemon mixture, remove, and sprinkle with salt. Once the grill is ready, put the potatoes on the grate. Cover the grill and cook for 3 to 6 minutes on each side. Remove the potatoes from the grill and serve hot.

*Makes 4 servings*

**Per serving:** 194 calories, 2 g protein, 11 g fat, 24 g carbohydrates

# SWEET POTATO FRIES

3    medium sweet potatoes (4 ounces each)

1    tablespoon extra-virgin olive oil

½    teaspoon salt

⅛    teaspoon black pepper

**MAKE IT**

Preheat the oven to 425°F.

Wash the potatoes well, leaving the skin on, and cut into quarters lengthwise.

Cut each quartered potato again lengthwise, making 3 wedges.

Toss the potatoes in the oil, salt, and pepper to coat them.

Bake until the potatoes are tender, about 45 minutes, turning them occasionally.

*Makes 4 servings*

**Per serving:** 105 calories, 5 g protein, 4 g fat, 17 g carbohydrates

# SWEET SAUTÉED CARROTS

5    whole carrots, sliced like coins

1    clove garlic, minced

1    tablespoon brown sugar

1    tablespoon low-sodium soy sauce

1    teaspoon Tabasco sauce (or to taste)

2    teaspoons extra-virgin olive oil

**MAKE IT**

Sauté all of the above ingredients until the carrots are crisp and tender.

*Makes 2 servings*

**Per serving:** 145 calories, 2 g protein, 8 g fat, 20 g carbohydrates

# MEDITERRANEAN-STYLE VEGETABLES

1   green bell pepper, chopped

1   zucchini, sliced

2   cloves garlic, minced

1   can (14.5 ounces) Italian stewed tomatoes

1   can (14.5 ounces) navy beans

2   teaspoons dried basil

2   teaspoons extra-virgin olive oil

6   tablespoons reduced-fat shredded Italian cheese blend

**MAKE IT**

Coat a large skillet with nonstick cooking spray.

Stir-fry the pepper, zucchini, and garlic over medium heat for about 5 minutes. Add the can of tomatoes.

Drain and rinse the beans. Add the basil to the beans, then add the mixture to the stir-fry. Bring to a boil. Reduce the heat and simmer for 10 minutes. Stir in the olive oil.

Sprinkle each serving with 2 tablespoons cheese.

*Makes 3 servings*

**Per serving:** 217 calories, 13 g protein, 5 g fat, 34 g carbohydrates

# SPINACH ORZO

½     bag (about 2 cups) frozen chopped spinach

1     can (14.5 ounces) Italian diced tomatoes

1     can (14.5 ounces) reduced-sodium chicken broth or water

½     package (about 8 ounces) dry whole wheat orzo pasta

4     ounces (½ bag) reduced-fat shredded Italian cheese blend

**MAKE IT**

Place the spinach in a medium saucepan over medium-high heat.

Add the can of tomatoes and the can of broth or water.

When the mixture comes to a boil, add the orzo.

Turn the heat down to medium and continue to cook for about 10 minutes (or until most liquid is absorbed), stirring constantly.

Stir in the shredded cheese.

*Makes 2 servings*

**Per serving:** 650 calories, 20 g protein, 12 g fat, 101 g carbohydrates

# SPICY MUSTARD SAUCE

1     teaspoon apple cider vinegar

1     teaspoon honey

1½   tablespoons spicy mustard

3     tablespoons reduced-fat olive oil mayonnaise

**MAKE IT**

Mix all the ingredients together in a small bowl. Use with salmon cakes (page 119) as a dipping sauce or on sandwiches or burgers as a condiment.

*Makes 5 tablespoons*

**Per serving (2 tablespoons):** 60 calories, 0 g protein, 4 g fat, 6 g carbohydrates

# SNACKS AND DESSERTS

## PEANUT BUTTER BALLS

½     cup peanut butter

1     tablespoon honey (local is best if you can find it
      at the store)

1     teaspoon vanilla extract

1–2 pinches of salt

1     tablespoon coconut flour (you can find this in the baking
      aisle at most grocery stores)

1–2 tablespoons dark mini chocolate chips

**MAKE IT**

In a medium bowl, mix together the peanut butter, honey, vanilla, and salt. Mix until smooth.

Add the coconut flour and stir. Fold in the chocolate chips. Using a large table-spoon, scoop out the mixture and roll into bite-size balls.

Place the balls into an airtight container and place into the freezer.

**Note:** You can keep these in the freezer up to 1 month.

*Makes 6 balls*

**Per serving (1 ball):** 51 calories, 1 g protein, 3 g fat, 6 g carbohydrates

# COTTAGE CHEESE SALAD

½   cup grapes

1   cup apple, chopped small

1   lettuce leaf

½   cup low-fat cottage cheese

**MAKE IT**

Wash the fruit and lettuce leaf. In a small bowl, stir together the cottage cheese and fruit.

Place in an airtight container overnight or use right away.

When ready to eat, place the mixture in the clean lettuce leaf.

*Makes 1 serving*

**Per serving:** 177 calories, 14 g protein, 3 g fat, 27 g carbohydrates


# COOKIE DOUGH YOGURT

1   tablespoon peanut butter

1   tablespoon dark mini chocolate chips

1   tablespoon sweetener (honey or blue agave)

¼   teaspoon vanilla extract

1   6-ounce cup vanilla light Greek yogurt

    Pinch of salt

**MAKE IT**

Combine all ingredients together in the yogurt cup or in a separate bowl. Mix well.

*Makes 1 serving*

**Per serving:** 284 calories, 15 g protein, 10 g fat, 38 g carbohydrates

# BAKED ZUCCHINI CHIPS

| | |
|---|---|
| 1 | **large zucchini** |
| ¼ | **cup whole grain bread crumbs, such as panko** |
| ¼ | **cup finely grated reduced-fat Parmesan cheese** |
| ¼ | **teaspoon black pepper** |
| ⅛ | **teaspoon cayenne pepper** |
| ⅛ | **teaspoon garlic powder** |
| | **Kosher or sea salt to taste** |
| 3 | **tablespoons fat-free milk** |

**MAKE IT**

Preheat the oven to 425°F.

Cut the zucchini into ⅛" to ¼" slices. In a small bowl, mix together all the dry ingredients.

Pour the milk into a small bowl. Dip the zucchini slices into the milk, then place the zucchini slices into the dry mixture to cover.

Coat a baking sheet with nonstick cooking spray and put the zucchini on the sheet. Bake for about 15 minutes.

Flip the chips over and continue baking until they are golden brown (about 15 minutes).

Allow the chips to cool, then place into a storage container.

*Makes 4 servings*

**Per serving:** 85 calories, 6 g protein, 4 g fat, 7 g carbohydrates

# BUFFALO CHICKEN AND POTATO WEDGES

2     sweet potatoes

1     egg white

1     teaspoon salt

½     teaspoon garlic powder

½     teaspoon black pepper

1     cup precooked rotisserie chicken (white meat only)

½     cup Buffalo sauce

½     cup reduced-fat shredded Cheddar cheese

      Optional: low-calorie ranch dressing for dipping

**MAKE IT**

Preheat the oven to 450°F.

Poke the potatoes with a fork and place them in the microwave for 2 minutes
to slightly soften them. Cut the potatoes into wedges and brush the wedges
with egg white. Place on a baking sheet covered with foil. Sprinkle the season-
ings over the potatoes. Bake until crisp, about 12 to 15 minutes.

In a small bowl, toss the chicken in with the Buffalo sauce.

Remove the potatoes from the oven and place the chicken and cheese on top
of the potatoes.

Return to the oven and bake for an additional 5 minutes.

If you like, drizzle low-calorie ranch dressing on top of the potatoes. The values
below do not include the ranch dressing.

*Makes 4 servings*

**Per serving:** 209 calories, 19 g protein, 8 g fat, 12 g carbohydrates

# MINI POPPERS

12   mini bell peppers
6   pieces low-fat string cheese

**MAKE IT**

Preheat the oven to broil.

Cut a vertical slit in each of the peppers, making sure to keep them intact.

Wash the peppers and remove all seeds.

Cut the string cheese in half and place the halves inside each of the peppers.

Cover a baking sheet with foil. Place the peppers on the sheet.

Broil the poppers until the cheese is melted, about 10 minutes.

*Makes 12 servings*

**Per serving:** 33 calories, 3 g protein, 1 g fat, 2 g carbohydrates

Only 2 ingredients, pal.
Doesn't get much easier!

# MOZZARELLA STICKS

12   sticks part-skim, reduced-sodium
     mozzarella string cheese

1    large egg, beaten

2    tablespoons flour

1    tablespoon dried parsley

2    teaspoons grated Parmesan cheese

¼    cup panko crumbs or Italian bread crumbs

    Olive oil cooking spray

**MAKE IT**

Cut the cheese sticks in half to make 24 pieces. Place the cheese in the freezer until frozen.

Beat the egg in a small bowl and set aside.

Put the flour in a separate bowl and set aside.

In a third bowl, combine the remaining dry ingredients.

**FOR ASSEMBLY-LINE PRODUCTION**

Place the frozen cheese in the flour and shake it off, then place it into the egg bowl.

Lastly, coat the cheese in the bread crumb mixture.

Place the sticks onto waxed paper until all cheese sticks are coated.

Put the cheese back into the freezer (at least 20 minutes) before baking. They must be frozen before baking.

Preheat your oven to 400°F.

Cover a baking sheet with foil, spray with olive oil spray, and place the sticks onto the baking sheet. Spray the sticks with olive oil.

Place the baking sheet toward the bottom of the oven and bake for 4 to 5 minutes.

Turn the sticks over and bake for an additional 4 to 5 minutes.

*Makes 24 pieces*

**Per serving (2 pieces):** 100 calories, 9 g protein, 7 g fat, 3 g carbohydrates

# CHOCOLATE CLOUD SANDWICHES

  1    container Cool Whip Lite (or other brand 95% fat-free
       whipped topping)
 14    chocolate graham crackers

**MAKE IT**

Allow the whipped topping to thaw slightly, enough so you can spoon it out.

Break the crackers in two.

Place 3 tablespoons of whipped topping in between two cracker halves, making 1 sandwich out of it.

Place the assembled crackers into an airtight container and freeze.

Freeze until the whipped topping is firm like an ice cream sandwich, approximately 3 hours.

*Makes 14 servings*

**Per serving (1 sandwich):** 90 calories, 1 g protein, 3 g fat, 17 g carbohydrates

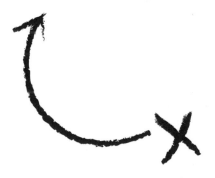

# BLACK BEAN DIP

1    can (15 ounces) black beans (drained/save juice)

½    teaspoon cayenne blend

2    teaspoons ground cumin

**MAKE IT**

In small bowl, mix together (with a hand mixer) the drained black beans, cayenne, and cumin.

Use the saved juice from the can to make the paste creamier. Add until you get the desired consistency.

*Makes 8 servings*

**Per serving (¼ cup):** 53 calories, 4 g protein, 0 g fat, 10 g carbohydrates


# SPICY ARTICHOKE DIP

1    can (8 ounces) artichoke hearts in water

¼    cup finely grated pepper jack cheese

1    teaspoon lemon juice

¾    cup reduced-fat olive oil mayonnaise

**MAKE IT**

Preheat the oven to 350°F.

Drain and chop the artichokes. Mix all the ingredients together.

Place in a shallow, ungreased 13″ x 9″ baking dish.

Bake until the mixture is bubbly, about 20 to 30 minutes.

Allow to cool and serve warm.

*Makes 16 servings*

**Per serving (2 tablespoons):** 39 calories, 1 g protein, 3 g fat, 2 g carbohydrates

# HUMMUS

1    **can (15 ounces) garbanzo beans**

2    **tablespoons lemon juice**

2    **tablespoons extra-virgin olive oil**

2    **teaspoons minced garlic**

**MAKE IT**

Drain the beans, keeping the liquid for later.

Place the beans and rest of the ingredients into a blender or food processor.

Process the ingredients for about 30 seconds.

Add the reserved bean liquid in small amounts until you get the desired consistency.

Chill and serve.

*Makes 8 servings*

**Per serving (¼ cup):** 90 calories, 3 g protein, 4 g fat, 10 g carbohydrates

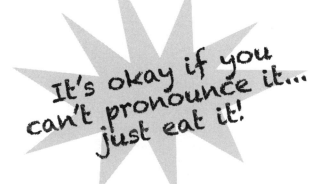

It's okay if you can't pronounce it... just eat it!

# CURRY DEVILED EGGS

| 8 | eggs |
|---|------|
| ¼ | cup reduced-fat mayonnaise |
| 2 | teaspoons Dijon or deli-style mustard |
| ¼ | teaspoon curry powder |

**MAKE IT**

Place a single layer of eggs in a saucepan of cold water. The water should cover the eggs by about 1 inch.

Bring the water to a boil on high heat. Cook for approximately 10 minutes.

Remove the eggs from the pan and crack them slightly by hitting them with a spoon.

Place the cracked eggs in cold water. Leave for 1 minute. Peel the eggs and cut lengthwise.

Remove the yolk from the eggs and place in a bowl. Smash with a fork.

Mix in the remaining ingredients and whisk until the mixture is smooth.

Place the mixture back into the eggs.

Cover and refrigerate until you're ready to eat.

*Makes 16 servings*

**Per serving (½ egg):** 48 calories, 3 g protein, 3 g fat, 1 g carbohydrates

# GET JUICED

A powerful juicer is a terrific cheat for the man who wants to boost his intake of antioxidants and other crucial nutrients without having to gnaw on bunches of carrots and kale. Buy the best blender/juicer that you can afford. The good ones typically come with a book of recipes for more than just beverages—even entire meals.

To get you going, I've included some of my favorite power-juice recipes and added a smoothie-builder cheat sheet to help you create your own concoctions.

Most of the juice recipes listed on the opposite page will yield between 16 and 20 ounces, depending on your juicer and how much of each ingredient you use. If you want to cut down on cleaning time, you can use a plastic grocery store bag and place it inside of the pulp collector. After you are done using the juicer, simply pull the bag out and toss the pulp into the trash can. This will greatly cut down on time and mess.

You can also double or triple the recipes and store the juice for later. You can safely keep the juice for about 3 days in a sealed container and it will retain its flavor. Some juices may separate after they sit a while, so you'll need to shake the juice up before pouring yourself another glass.

Depending on your juicer, you may need to cut, core, and/or remove the outer skin of your produce. Make sure to thoroughly clean all your produce before juicing.

# BEET THIS

| | |
|---|---|
| 2 | beets |
| 1 | large carrot |
| 3 | celery stalks |
| ½ | cucumber |
| 1 | finger ginger |
| ½ | medium green apple |

# MEAN JOE GREEN

| | |
|---|---|
| 1 | finger ginger |
| 4 | celery stalks |
| 2 | medium green apples |
| 1 | bunch kale |
| ½ | lemon |

# ONE HOT MAMA

| | |
|---|---|
| 1 | bunch cilantro |
| 2 | large cucumbers |
| 1 | lime |
| | Coconut water, to taste (Mix into juice after you are done juicing the vegetables.) |

# ORANGE YOU AWAKE?

| | |
|---|---|
| 3 | carrots |
| 1 | medium green apple |
| 1 | lime (rind removed) |
| 1 | orange (rind removed) |

# PEARFECT

| | |
|---|---|
| 1 | cup fresh basil |
| 1 | finger ginger |
| 1 | orange |
| 2 | pears |
| 4 | cups spinach |

# SLIM JIM

| | |
|---|---|
| ½ | large cucumber |
| 1 | grapefruit |
| 1 | medium green apple |
| 1 | bunch kale |
| 1 | lime |

# TURN UP THE HEAT

| | |
|---|---|
| 2 | stalks celery |
| ½ | bunch cilantro |
| 1 | large cucumber |
| 1 | clove garlic |
| 2 | stalks celery |
| ½ | jalapeño (seeded) |
| ½ | lemon |
| ½ | onion |
| ½ | head romaine lettuce |

# WHAT'S UP, DOC?

| | |
|---|---|
| 2 | medium green apples |
| 3 | carrots |
| 1 | finger ginger |
| ½ | lemon |

# Build the Perfect Smoothie Cheat Sheet

When building your smoothie, remember to watch the calorie content of the items you're tossing into your blender. The more items, the higher the calories. If you use frozen fruit, you can cut down on the amount of ice you need to add to your smoothie. To construct a great meal replacement, select one item from each step below, dump, and hit blend.

## 1. Choose a Base

Add 1 to 2 cups:

Almond milk
Coconut milk
Coconut water
Fat-free milk
Fruit juice
Iced coffee
Iced green tea
Rice milk
Soy milk
Water

## 2. Add Fruit and/or Vegetables

Choose 2, fresh or frozen:

Apple
Banana
Beet
Berries
Cherries
Kale
Kiwifruit
Mango
Peach
Pear
Pineapple
Spinach
Watermelon

## 3. Add a Thickener and Protein

Chia seeds
Cottage cheese (low fat)
Frozen yogurt (low fat)
Oats
Peanut butter (or other nut butter)
Protein powder
Yogurt

## 4. Flavor It or Sweeten It Up (optional)

Add to your taste:

Agave
Almond extract
Basil
Cinnamon
Honey
Mint
Nutmeg
Splenda
Stevia
Vanilla extract

## 5. Give It a Nutrition Power Boost

Fish oil
Ground flaxseed
Probiotic
Unsweetened cocoa powder
Wheatgrass

# DINE OUT AND STILL WIN!

Sometimes you find yourself at a restaurant for a meal with family or friends and, well, it would just be rude to sit outside in the car; cold, too, in the dead of winter. You can dine out and still destroy your competition if you keep an eye on your calories in these dens of over-indulgence. This calorie cheat sheet of the fare at some popular restaurants will help, or simply ask the server for a nutrition listing for their menu items.

### Applebee's (all under 550 calories)

Napa Chicken & Portobellos

Roasted Garlic Sirloin

Signature Sirloin with Garlic Herb Shrimp

Zesty Roma Chicken & Shrimp

### Au Bon Pain

½ Turkey & Swiss Sandwich, 370

Apple Cinnamon Oatmeal (small), 190

Egg Whites & Cheddar Breakfast Sandwich, 230

Egg Whites, Cheddar & Avocado Breakfast Sandwich, 310

Meat Lasagna, 470

Veggie Soup (large), 240

Whole Wheat Skinny Bagel, 90

### Bob Evans

Apple Cranberry Spinach Salad, 372

Be Fit Breakfast, 352

Grilled Chicken Breast, 446

Grilled Salmon Fillet, 408

Turkey Sausage Breakfast, 340

Veggie Omelet, 310

### California Pizza Kitchen

Asparagus & Arugula Salad, 190

Dakota Smashed Pea & Barley Soup (cup), 170

Fire Roasted Chile Relleno, 380

Sedona Tortilla Soup (cup), 270

## Carl's Jr.

Big Hamburger, 216

Charbroiled Chicken Club, 264

Famous Star with cheese, 286

Sourdough Breakfast Sandwich, 200

## Chili's

Grilled Chicken Salad, 430

Lighter Choice Classic Sirloin (6 ounces), 250

Lighter Choice Grilled Salmon, 580

Mango Chile Chicken, 580

Mango Chile Tilapia, 620

Sweet & Spicy Chicken, 580

## Chipotle

Burrito with chicken, fajita veggies, and green tomatillo salsa, 515

Burrito bowl with chicken, fajita veggies, guacamole, and red tomatillo salsa, 400

## Denny's

2 Egg Whites, 50

Fit Fare Chicken Avocado Sandwich, 490

Fit Fare Omelet, 350

Fit Fare Veggie Skillet, 330

Fit Slam, 360

Hearty Wheat Pancakes (2), 310

## Dunkin' Donuts

Bacon, Egg & Cheese English Muffin, 290

English Muffin, 140

## Jason's Deli

Mediterranean Wrap (without sides), 320

Savory Chicken Salad Wrap (without sides), 350

Spinach Veggie Wrap, 350

Turkey Wrap (without sides), 410

## LongHorn Steakhouse

Flo's Filet (7 ounces), 430

Grilled Rainbow Trout, 380

7 Pepper Sirloin, half salad (lunch menu), 260

Sierra Chicken (lighter portion), 340

## Noodles & Company

Bangkok Curry (small), 260

Curry Soup (small), 230

Indonesian Peanut Sauté (small), 420

The Med Sandwich, 330

## Olive Garden

Capellini Pomodoro without protein, 490 (dinner portion), 480 (lunch portion)

Herb Grilled Salmon, 480

Ravioli di Portobello (lunch portion), 450

Seafood Brodetto, 480

Venetian Apricot Chicken, 400 (dinner portion), 290 (lunch portion)

## Panera Bread

Breakfast Power with Ham on Whole Grain, 340

Steel Cut Oatmeal with Strawberries & Pecans, 340

## Red Lobster

Asparagus, 60

Bar Harbor Salad with shrimp (no dressing), 420

Broccoli, 40

Green Beans, 50

Rock Lobster Tail, 210

Veggie Medley, 40

Wood Grilled Fresh Salmon (half portion), 290

Wood Grilled Rainbow Trout (half portion), 200

Wood Grilled Tilapia (half portion), 190

## Romano's Macaroni Grill (all under 600 calories)

Caprese

Grilled Chicken Spiedini

Grilled Shrimp Spiedini

Mediterranean Sea Bass

Pollo Caprese

Warm Spinach & Shrimp

## Ruby Tuesday

Hickory Bourbon Chicken Fit & Trim, 355

Jumbo Crab Cake Fit & Trim, 270

Petite Chicken Fresco Fit & Trim, 396

Petite Sirloin Fit & Trim, 354

Sliced Tomatoes with Balsamic Vinaigrette Fit & Trim, 52

Spaghetti Squash Marinara Fit & Trim, 260

## Starbucks

Caramel Frappuccino Light (drink), 130

Fruit Cup, 90

Iced Skinny Latte (drink), 60

Nonfat Caffé Latte (drink), 100

Nonfat Caramel Macchiato (drink), 140

Shaken Tazo Iced Black Tea Lemonade (drink), 100

Spinach, Roasted Tomato, Feta & Egg White Wrap, 280

Strawberry Blueberry Yogurt Parfait, 300

Turkey Bacon, Egg White, and Cheddar Breakfast Sandwich, 320

## Taco Bell

Bacon Egg Burrito, 156

Bean Burrito, 198

Burrito Supreme Chicken, 240

Cantina Bowl Chicken or Steak, 415

Chicken Burrito, 169

Chicken Soft Taco, 92

Steak and Egg Burrito, 163

# Eat with Your Hands

A quick way to eyeball proper serving sizes so you won't overeat by accident.

| SIZE | FOOD | CALORIES |
|---|---|---|
| **Fist = 1 cup** | Fruit | 75 |
| | Rice | 200 |
| | Veggies | 40 |
| **Palm = 3 ounces** | Fish | 160 |
| | Meat | 160 |
| | Poultry | 160 |
| **Handful = 1 ounce** | Nuts | 170 |
| | Raisins | 85 |
| **2 handfuls = 1 ounce** | Chips | 150 |
| | Popcorn | 120 |
| | Pretzels | 100 |
| **Thumb = 1 ounce** | Hard cheese | 100 |
| | Peanut butter | 170 |
| **Thumb tip = 1 teaspoon** | Cooking oil | 40 |
| | Mayo/butter | 30 |
| | Sugar | 15 |

It's all about portion control

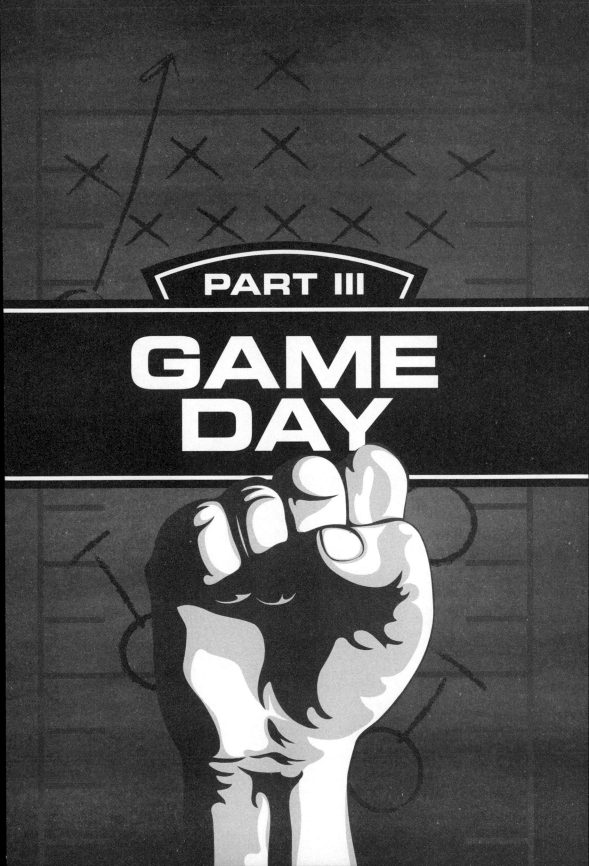

# PART III

# GAME DAY

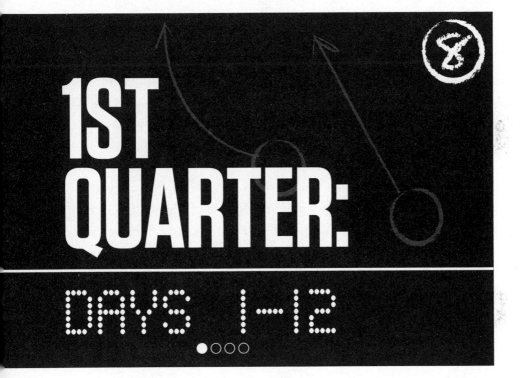

# 1ST QUARTER:

## DAYS 1-12

●○○○

**YOU CAN'T WIN THE CONTEST DURING THE FIRST QUARTER, BUT YOU CAN SURE AS HELL LOSE IT.** Don't be an overachiever during this quarter; just follow the plan. No Hail Mary passes here; just get your feet wet and build up your base fitness for the later quarters. Eat clean and keep a good attitude.

On page 163, you'll find a schedule that shows your workouts for each day in this 12-day quarter. A little later in the chapter, you'll see your first-quarter meal plan and a shopping list that'll make it easy to get all the groceries you need to follow the meal plan. Each of the menus in this 60-day plan is designed to meet minimum daily needs for fruits, vegetables, fiber, omega-3 fatty acids, and calcium/vitamin D. They provide ample protein for the individual following a low-calorie diet for weight loss but trying to maintain muscle mass. They are low in saturated fat and low in added sugars. Inevitably there may be food combinations you have never tried. Be adventurous and give them a shot. Keep track of foods you like. You can try more new foods and collect more favorites with each of the following quarter menus. You will also notice that there are a few meatless days. Stop sniveling. I did this to encourage you to try more plant-based proteins, which is proven to reduce cardiovascular disease and increase longevity. So suck it up!

If you feel like you must consume alcoholic beverages, use your after-dinner snack calories for your drink instead of consuming the listed snack. Keep in mind that one light beer is about 100 calories, or the caloric equivalent of 4 ounces of wine, or $1\frac{1}{2}$ ounces of hard liquor. Also see "Don't Party Yourself out of the Running" on page 193.

It's time to work. As described in the Chapter 4, your workouts are made up of Rival Strength Challenges, Functional Stability Workouts, HIIT Workouts, and Cardio. Here's how they play out.

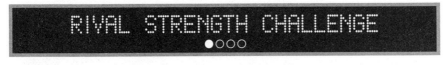

RIVAL STRENGTH CHALLENGE

# 747

**Goal: Perform as many rounds as possible in 15 minutes.**

**Equipment: Stopwatch or clock with second hand**

Complete all the required reps before moving on to the next exercise. Focus on quality reps. When you finish with the last pushup, jump back into squats. Rest as needed, but remember you are being timed.

- 7 Squats
- 4 Burpees
- 7 Pushups

*Note:* The exercise descriptions and photographs are found in Chapter 5.

RIVAL STRENGTH CHALLENGE

# 20 MINUTES IN HELL

**Goal: Perform as many rounds as possible in 20 minutes.**

**Equipment: Stopwatch or clock with second hand**

Complete all the required reps before moving on to the next exercise. Focus on quality reps. When you finish with the last squat, jump back into mountain climbers. Rest as needed, but remember you are being timed.

- 5 Mountain Climbers
- 10 Pushups
- 15 Squats

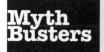
**Myth Busters**

## You Have to Work Out with Machines to Get a Great Workout

This is absolute rubbish. In most cases, you can get a superior training session using solely your own body weight and/or a set of dumbbells. Did the Romans or the Spartans have a leg press or a chest press machine? I don't think so . . . and you don't need them either.

One of the major downsides to machines, other than the fact that you have to belong to a gym to use them, is that they keep you locked into a single position. Why is this bad? Well, they don't allow you to perform movements that we perform during everyday life, as well as on the court or field.

Your body moves in three planes: sagittal, frontal, and transverse. At any given time, your body is capable of producing movements in all three directions. However, when using an exercise machine, more often than not you are in a fixed position, thus only working one plane.

So why is multiplane movement important?

- The body/muscles get worked from multiple angles.
- You work smaller stabilizer muscles.
- You recruit more muscle activation from secondary muscles.
- It helps decrease your risk of injury in everyday life and during sports/activity.
- Put simply, you get more bang for your buck.

# FUNCTIONAL STABILITY WORKOUT #1

●○○○

Do each of the exercises in the order listed below. Complete all sets before moving on to the next exercise. Rest as needed. For exercise photos and descriptions, see Chapter 5.

| EXERCISE | SETS / REPS |
|---|---|
| Crunch | 2 / 15 |
| Single-Leg Bridge | 2 / 10 (each leg; hold each rep for 5 seconds) |
| Single-Leg Drop | 2 / 10 (each leg) |
| Bird Dog | 2 / 10 (each side) |
| Plank | 3 / 1 (hold each for 20 seconds) |
| Squat with Arms Up | 3 / 8 |
| Seated Russian Twist | 3 / 15 (twisting left and right = 1 rep) |

Want more?
Then doubledown
with a bonus cardio
workout on page 203

HIIT WORKOUT

●○○○

# VALOR

**Goal: Complete three rounds.**

**Equipment: Stopwatch or clock with second hand**

Perform all exercises in the sequence shown below. Do each move for 20 seconds, rest for 40 seconds, and then move to the next exercise. Do the circuit a total of three times in 15 minutes.

Jumping Jacks

Mountain Climbers

Jump Rope

High Knees

Side-to-Side Jumps

Do it. Then Log it!

# 1ST QUARTER WORKOUT SCHEDULE

●○○○

**Day 1:** Rival Strength Challenge: 747 (page 159)

**Day 2:** Functional Stability Workout #1 (page 161)

**Day 3:** HIIT Workout: Valor (opposite page)

**Day 4:** Cardio

**Day 5:** Rival Strength Challenge: 20 Minutes in Hell (page 159)

**Day 6:** Functional Stability Workout #1

**Day 7:** HIIT Workout: Valor

**Day 8:** Cardio

**Day 9:** Rival Strength Challenge: 747

**Day 10:** Functional Stability Workout #1

**Day 11:** HIIT Workout: Valor

**Day 12:** Cardio

*Note:* You can do extra cardio every day, and as often as you would like. See the bonus cardio workouts beginning on page 203.

## LOG IT

Mark off each daily task as you complete it.

**WOD** = Workout of the day

**H₂0** = Drink 12 glasses of water

**MFP** = Logged on MyFitnessPal

| DAY 1 | DAY 2 | DAY 3 | DAY 4 | DAY 5 | DAY 6 |
|---|---|---|---|---|---|
| ☐WOD ☐H₂0 ☐MFP | ☐WOD ☐H₂0 ☐MFP | ☐WOD ☐H₂0 ☐MFP | ☐WOD ☐H₂0 ☐MFP | ☐WOD ☐H₂0 ☐MFP | ☐WOD ☐H₂0 ☐MFP |

| DAY 7 | DAY 8 | DAY 9 | DAY 10 | DAY 11 | DAY 12 |
|---|---|---|---|---|---|
| ☐WOD ☐H₂0 ☐MFP | ☐WOD ☐H₂0 ☐MFP | ☐WOD ☐H₂0 ☐MFP | ☐WOD ☐H₂0 ☐MFP | ☐WOD ☐H₂0 ☐MFP | ☐WOD ☐H₂0 ☐MFP |

# 1ST QUARTER SHOPPING LIST

●○○○

# (DAYS 1-12)

Here's everything you need to make the meals listed in this quarter's menu:

## PRODUCE

5 fruits of choice
(1 cup or 1 piece = 1 fruit choice)

5 apples
(1 green apple + 4 others of choice)

3 bananas or 3 more apples

1 carton blueberries

1 carton strawberries

1 carton berries of choice

3 cups cut mixed fruit

1 cup cut pineapple rings

3 limes

3 lemons

4 large ripe avocados

1 bag clementines

3 bags fresh baby spinach

1 bag salad greens

1 bag coleslaw mix
(shredded cabbage and carrots)

3 large onions

6 cloves garlic

1 bag baby carrots

1 bag snap peas

1 bag celery sticks

1 red bell pepper

1 bag snow peas

5 whole carrots

2 tomatoes

1 plum tomato

1 bunch broccoli

1 bunch broccolini

1 bunch asparagus

1 bunch cilantro

2 pounds sweet potatoes

8 small pieces sushi rolls (you should eat this within 2 days of purchasing it to ensure optimal freshness)

4 nigiri sushi (you should eat this within 2 days of purchasing it to ensure optimal freshness)

## DELI

6 ounces reduced-sodium turkey lunch meat

1 package turkey bacon

1 rotisserie chicken

## BAKERY

1 loaf whole wheat bread
(like Nature's Own)

1 package Mission Carb Balance tortillas

1 package whole wheat naan
(like Stonefire)

1 package whole wheat hamburger buns

## MEAT

11 ounces 95% lean ground beef

2 pounds pork tenderloin

1 pound chicken tenderloins

4 chicken breasts

4 ounces salmon fillet

## DAIRY

18 eggs or 3 cartons pasteurized egg whites

1 package reduced-fat cheese slices

3 cups (6 ounces each) 0% Greek yogurt of choice + 1 cup (6 ounces) vanilla 0% Greek yogurt

1 gallon 1% sweet acidophilus or fat-free milk

1 tub low-fat cottage cheese

1 tub low-fat sour cream

1 package low-fat string cheese

1 bag reduced-fat Italian shredded cheese blend

1 package grated Parmesan cheese

1 bag reduced-fat Mexican shredded cheese blend

1 bag reduced-fat pepper jack shredded cheese

1 tub Smart Balance Light butter spread

1 container fresh Buitoni whole wheat cheese tortellini

1 tub basil-garlic pesto sauce

## FROZEN FOODS

Vitalicious Vita-Egg breakfast sandwiches (if not making your own)

1 box Kashi Blueberry Waffles

1 bag roasted red potatoes

1 bag green beans

1 bag (15 ounces) whole kernel corn

2 containers Cool Whip Lite (or other brand 95% fat-free whipped topping)

1 bag (26–30 count) shrimp, cooked, peeled, deveined

## SHELF GOODS

1 bottle Dijon or spicy mustard

1 tube prepared wasabi

1 jar reduced-fat olive oil mayonnaise

1 jar hot sauce (like Tabasco)

1 bottle low-fat salad dressing

1 bottle barbecue sauce

1 bottle reduced-sodium soy sauce

1 jar marinara sauce (like Ragú Light)

1 jar dill pickles

1 jar (8 ounces) artichoke hearts, packed in water

1 can diced tomatoes

3 cans black beans

1 can garbanzo beans (or chickpeas)

1 can baked beans

1 can crabmeat

1 can medium shrimp

1 foil pouch (2.6 ounces) tuna, packed in water

3 small cans mandarin oranges, packed in juice

1 bag dried cherries (just cherries, no added sugar or preservatives)

2 boxes Imagine or Pacific soup

1 box (32 ounces) reduced-sodium chicken broth

1 can Campbell's 98% Fat-Free Cream of Chicken soup

1 bag brown rice

1 package Minute Brown and Wild Rice cups

1 box whole wheat spaghetti (like Ronzoni Healthy Harvest)

1 bag sliced almonds

1 bag dark cocoa–dusted almonds

1 bag sunflower seed kernels

1 bag dark mini chocolate chips

1 bottle pure maple syrup

1 bottle honey

1 jar natural jam (like Polaner)

1 jar nut butter (like Peter Pan Reduced Fat Peanut Butter)

1 packet taco seasoning

Jerk seasoning

Crushed red pepper

Ground cumin

Ground cinnamon

Salt

Ground black pepper

1 bottle extra-virgin olive oil

1 bottle apple cider vinegar

1 box sweetener packets
(if desired, like Splenda or Truvia)

1 bag brown sugar

1 box sugar-free hot chocolate mix

1 box old-fashioned oats (or 1 box Quaker Weight Control Instant Oatmeal if not making your own)

1 box Kashi GO LEAN original cereal or 1 box Special K Protein cereal

1 box original Cheerios

1 bag Bob's Red Mill Muesli

1 box chocolate graham crackers

1 box Pepperidge Farms Four-Cheese Cheese Crisps

1 box microwave popcorn, 100-calorie bags

8 ounces diet root beer

IST QUARTER MEAL PLAN
●○○○

A quick reminder that all four quarters and the overtime menus are based on approximately 2,000 calories per day. Depending on your personal metabolic requirements, you may need to adjust your daily calories to reflect your personal needs. You might want to go back and review the information in Chapter 6. If you skipped over the caloric-calculating formulas on page 96, go back and do it now. If you were planning to log your food and workouts on MyFitnessPal and haven't yet set up your account, do that now as well. Their system will automatically calculate your daily caloric requirements for you.

On page 181 in the Get More Calories Cheat Sheet, you will find quick ways to add anywhere from 25 to 100 calories to your daily intake. Otherwise you can easily cut or add to your portion sizes from our recipes.

**Example: Mozzarella Sticks (page 141):
serving size = 2 pieces (100 calories).**

**To add 100 calories, double up your portion
by eating 4 pieces (200 calories).**

**To cut 50 calories from your daily intake,
eat only 1 piece (50 calories).**

If your caloric needs are dramatically less than 2,000 calories per day, I suggest that you distribute the deficit throughout your meals. Cutting them out all at once could lead to feeling hungry and deprived.

Now go eat clean and train dirty! This first quarter sets the tone for the whole game.

*Note:* If you have leftovers and do not see them on the menu in the following 4 days, freeze them for ease and convenience at a later date.

# Day 1

### BREAKFAST

1 breakfast sandwich (2 slices whole wheat toast, 3 cooked egg whites, 1 slice reduced-fat cheese, 1 slice turkey bacon)

1 fruit choice

(or you can substitute 2 Vitalicious Vita-Egg breakfast sandwiches + 1 fruit choice)

### LUNCH

2 cups **Black Beans and Rice** (page 126)

### SNACK

1 banana or apple

1½ tablespoons nut butter

### DINNER

6 ounces rotisserie chicken breast

2½ cups **Fruit and Almond Salad** (page 116)

### SNACK

1 cup sliced strawberries

4 tablespoons Cool Whip Lite

1 tablespoon dark mini chocolate chips

# Day 2

### BREAKFAST

¾ cup old-fashioned oats cooked in 1 cup milk + water

1 apple, chopped, added to oats

1 teaspoon Splenda + 1 teaspoon cinnamon

2 tablespoons sliced almonds

(or 2 packs Quaker Weight Control Instant Oatmeal + 1 fruit choice)

### LUNCH

2 slices whole wheat bread

3 ounces turkey lunch meat

2 teaspoons reduced-fat olive oil mayo or spicy mustard

1 slice reduced-fat cheese

1 fruit choice

20 Pepperidge Farms Four-Cheese Cheese Crisps

### SNACK

15 baby carrots

15 snap peas

¼ cup **Hummus** (page 144)

### DINNER

5 ounces rotisserie chicken breast

1½ cups roasted red potatoes

1½ cups fresh baby spinach sautéed in garlic

1 cup **Sweet Sautéed Carrots** (page 133) (or frozen glazed baby carrots)

### SNACK

2 **Chocolate Cloud Sandwiches** (page 142)

# Day 3

## BREAKFAST

1 breakfast sandwich (2 slices whole wheat toast, 3 cooked egg whites, 1 slice reduced-fat cheese, 1 slice turkey bacon)

1 fruit choice

(or you can substitute 2 Vitalicious Vita-Egg breakfast sandwiches + 1 fruit choice)

## LUNCH

2 cups **Black Beans and Rice** (page 126)

## SNACK

1 cup (6 ounces) 0% Greek yogurt

3 clementines

## DINNER

1 piece whole wheat naan

½ cup marinara sauce

¼ cup reduced-fat Italian shredded cheese blend

(make pizza using ingredients above)

Side salad of 3 cups fresh baby spinach or other salad greens, 2 slices crumbled turkey bacon, 2 tablespoons low-fat salad dressing

## SNACK

1 tablespoon dark mini chocolate chips

¼ cup dried cherries

# Day 4

## BREAKFAST

¾ cup old-fashioned oats cooked in 1 cup milk + water

1 apple, chopped, added to oats

1 teaspoon Splenda + 1 teaspoon cinnamon

1 tablespoon sliced almonds

(or 2 packs Quaker Weight Control Instant Oatmeal + 1 fruit choice)

## LUNCH

2 cups Imagine or Pacific soup

½ piece whole wheat naan

## SNACK

1 banana or apple

1½ tablespoons nut butter

## DINNER

1½ cups whole wheat spaghetti (dry noodles with the diameter of a quarter)

¾ cup marinara sauce

3 ounces 95% lean ground beef, browned, added to sauce

3 cups salad greens

2 tablespoons low-fat salad dressing

2 tablespoons reduced-fat Italian shredded cheese blend

## SNACK

2 **Chocolate Cloud Sandwiches** (page 142)

## Day 5

### BREAKFAST

1 breakfast sandwich (2 slices whole wheat toast, 3 cooked egg whites, 1 slice reduced-fat cheese, 1 slice turkey bacon)

1 fruit choice

(or you can substitute 2 Vitalicious Vita-Egg breakfast sandwiches + 1 fruit choice)

### LUNCH

2 slices whole wheat bread

3 ounces turkey lunch meat

2 teaspoons reduced-fat olive oil mayo or spicy mustard

1 slice reduced-fat cheese

1 fruit choice

20 Pepperidge Farm Four-Cheese Cheese Crisps

### SNACK

15 baby carrots

15 snap peas

¼ cup **Hummus** (page 144)

### DINNER

1 95% lean ground beef patty (4 ounces)

1 whole wheat hamburger bun

1 cup steamed green beans

⅔ cup baked beans

Lettuce, tomato, and mustard

1 slice reduced-fat cheese on patty

### SNACK

1 tablespoon dark mini chocolate chips

¼ cup dried cherries

## Day 6

### BREAKFAST

2 Kashi Blueberry Waffles

1 cup berries

1 tablespoon honey or pure maple syrup

1 cup cooked egg whites

1 slice reduced-fat cheese in eggs

### LUNCH

1 95% lean ground beef patty (4 ounces)

1 slice reduced-fat cheese on patty

1 cup steamed green beans

⅔ cup baked beans

### SNACK

¼ cup **Spicy Artichoke Dip** (page 143)

20 baby carrots

10 celery sticks

### DINNER

4 nigiri sushi

4 spicy tuna rolls (small pieces)

4 California rolls (small pieces)

1 tablespoon reduced-sodium soy sauce

1 tablespoon wasabi

### SNACK

1 cup sliced strawberries

4 tablespoons Cool Whip Lite

1 tablespoon dark mini chocolate chips

# 5 Surefire Ways to Sabotage Yourself

1. **Underestimate how many calories you are consuming.** You must expend more energy (calories) than you take in to lose weight, period. If you don't, you won't lose weight and you won't win. How do you know if you are eating the right amount of food to lose weight? You keep track of your eating. Yes, that means counting calories. Sure, you can guess, and you're likely to be wrong! The average person underestimates their daily calories by as much as 600 per day.

2. **Overestimate how many calories you are burning.** The best way to know for sure how many calories you are burning off is to either (a) wear a heart rate monitor that calculates calories burned or (b) log your workouts onto a system like MyFitnessPal. But I really like option (c): Do both! Wear a heart rate monitor that calculates your calories and log them into your online or handwritten daily journal.

3. **Don't get enough sleep.** Research in the *American Journal of Human Biology* suggests that people with shorter sleep cycles (and who might be sleep deprived) have a higher BMI (body mass index) than those who get adequate sleep. Why is this? Researchers believe that sleep deprivation increases levels of a hormone called ghrelin, which signals that the body is hungry. On the flip side, it decreases leptin, which signals that the body is full. Not to mention that since you're dragging throughout the day, you are more likely to eat sugar-filled foods to try to get you over a midday slump. Lack of sleep can also lead to skipping workouts because you're too tired. Now if you are waking up a bit earlier to exercise, that's a good thing, but just make sure you are getting enough sleep so that you have the energy and motivation to get your workout in.

4. **Binge on healthy foods.** Just because something is healthy doesn't make it *calorie free*. Actually some healthy foods and snacks like granola and avocados are quite calorie dense. So with that in mind, go back and reread number one on this list again. Track your calories.

5. **Mistake thirst for hunger.** Are you really hungry, or do you just need something to drink? This is a question you should ask yourself before stuffing your face with food. Mild dehydration can trigger feelings of hunger. When you stay hydrated, your appetite decreases because your body is getting what it needs (hydration); thus, you maintain a feeling of being satisfied. So try chugging a big glass of water before each meal or when you find yourself craving things you know you shouldn't be eating.

# Day 7

**BREAKFAST**

5 egg whites (omelet)

1 cup broccoli

1 plum tomato, diced

¼ cup reduced-fat shredded cheese

2 slices whole wheat toast with 1 tablespoon natural jam

**LUNCH**

2 cups Imagine or Pacific soup

½ piece whole wheat naan

**SNACK**

¼ cup **Spicy Artichoke Dip** (page 143)

20 baby carrots

10 celery sticks

**DINNER**

¾ cup **Easy Pulled Pork** (page 123)

1 whole wheat bun

1½ cups shredded cabbage + 1½ tablespoons reduced-fat olive oil mayo, salt/black pepper, 1 teaspoon apple cider vinegar

1 sliced apple, microwaved with 1 teaspoon cinnamon and sugar

(freeze leftover pork in portioned-out containers for future use, as well as buns)

**SNACK**

2 **Chocolate Cloud Sandwiches** (page 142)

# Day 8

**BREAKFAST**

2 cups Kashi GO LEAN original cereal

1 cup berries

1¼ cups fat-free milk

**LUNCH**

1 serving **Crab-Baked Avocados** (page 125)

1 cup coleslaw mix with 1 tablespoon reduced-fat olive oil mayo, 1 teaspoon cider vinegar, salt/black pepper

**SNACK**

1 banana or apple

1½ tablespoons nut butter

**DINNER**

6 ounces shrimp (cooked, peeled)

½ cup mandarin oranges

1 large red bell pepper, chopped (roasted if desired)

1 cup steamed snow peas

3 tablespoons low-fat salad dressing

1 cup Minute Brown and Wild Rice

**SNACK**

8 ounces sugar-free hot chocolate made with 8 ounces fat-free milk

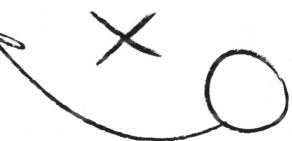

# Day 9

### BREAKFAST

1 cup (6 ounces) 0% Greek yogurt

1½ cups mixed fruit

¼ cup Bob's Red Mill Muesli

1 slice whole wheat toast with 1 teaspoon Smart Balance Light butter spread

### LUNCH

1 serving **Crab-Baked Avocados** (page 125)

1 cup coleslaw mix with 1 tablespoon reduced-fat olive oil mayo, 1 teaspoon cider vinegar, salt/black pepper

### SNACK

1 cup mandarin oranges, juice drained

¾ cup low-fat cottage cheese

1 tablespoon sunflower kernels

### DINNER

1½ cups fresh Buitoni whole wheat cheese tortellini

2 cups fresh baby spinach

1 tablespoon basil-garlic pesto sauce

1 tablespoon grated Parmesan cheese

### SNACK

1 cup Cheerios

8 ounces fat-free milk

# Day 10

### BREAKFAST

2 cups Kashi GO LEAN original cereal

1 cup berries

1¼ cups fat-free milk

### LUNCH

1 cup fresh Buitoni whole wheat cheese tortellini

2 cups fresh baby spinach

1 tablespoon basil-garlic pesto sauce

1 tablespoon grated Parmesan cheese

### SNACK

1 cup mandarin oranges, juice drained

¾ cup low-fat cottage cheese

1 tablespoon sunflower kernels

### LUNCH

2 servings **Fix and Forget Enchilada Soup** (page 118)

¼ cup reduced-fat Mexican shredded cheese blend

2 tablespoons low-fat sour cream

2 Mission Carb Balance tortillas (cut each into 4 pieces, spray with cooking spray, and toast in oven @ 400°F until crisp; about 6 to 7 minutes)

(freeze ¾ of soup for future weeks)

### SNACK

20 dark cocoa–dusted almonds

# WORKOUT WAR MVP

# JIM O'CONNOR

| | | | |
|---|---|---|---|
| **AGE:** | 27 | **% WEIGHT LOSS:** | 10.47% |
| **OCCUPATION:** | Executive chef | **% BODY FAT LOST:** | 10.9% |
| **STARTING WEIGHT:** | 236.8 | **FAT MASS LOST:** | −30.8 pounds |
| **ENDING WEIGHT:** | 212 | **LEAN MASS GAINED:** | +6 pounds |
| **ACTUAL LBS LOST:** | 24.8 | **COMBO % LOST:** | 21.37% |

## Game Recap

Jim dropped his body fat by almost 11 percent while gaining 6 pounds of muscle to destroy his opponents in the Workout War pilot program I conducted last year at my gym in Tennessee. Nobody could touch him. Jim believes the competition aspect of the program lit the fire under his ass to work crazy hard. "I knew the only way to be successful and win was to be extremely disciplined and focused," he says. "I kept on telling myself, 'There is always going to be someone training as hard, if not harder, than you.'"

But his motivation was more than winning the cash kitty. "You're invested, more than just the money aspect. It's like I'm committed and I want to win for myself," he says.

Once Jim started seeing results, he started pushing himself even further. "I didn't think I could do it in the beginning, but once I was in, I was like, 'I can do this,' and seeing the results really keeps you going."

# Day 11

### BREAKFAST

1 cup (6 ounces) 0% Greek yogurt

1½ cups mixed fruit

¼ cup Bob's Red Mill Muesli

1 slice whole wheat toast with 1 teaspoon Smart Balance Light butter spread

### LUNCH

2 servings **Fix and Forget Enchilada Soup** (page 118)

¼ cup reduced-fat Mexican shredded cheese blend

2 tablespoons low-fat sour cream

1 Mission Carb Balance tortilla (cut into 4 pieces, spray with cooking spray, and toast in oven @ 400°F until crisp; about 6–7 minutes)

### SNACK

1 apple or banana

1½ tablespoons nut butter

### DINNER

4 ounces poached salmon

1½ cups asparagus

2 cups roasted red potatoes

2 tablespoons **Spicy Mustard Sauce** (page 135)

### SNACK

1 bag 100-calorie microwave popcorn

4 tablespoons grated Parmesan cheese + black pepper (added to popcorn)

# Day 12

### BREAKFAST

2 cups Kashi GO LEAN original cereal

1 cup berries

1¼ cups fat-free milk

### LUNCH

1 Mission Carb Balance tortilla

1 foil pouch water-packed tuna

1 tablespoon reduced-fat olive oil mayo

1 pickle, cut into pieces

1 tablespoon mustard

1 cup fresh baby spinach

(make wrap of above)

3 clementines

20 almonds, your choice of flavor

### SNACK

1 bag 100-calorie microwave popcorn

2 pieces low-fat string cheese

### DINNER

1 serving **Grilled Jerk Chicken** (page 123)

1 serving **Grilled Sweet Potatoes** (page 132)

1 cup broccolini, steamed

1 cup grilled pineapple rings

### SNACK

1 tablespoon dark mini chocolate chips

¼ cup dried cherries

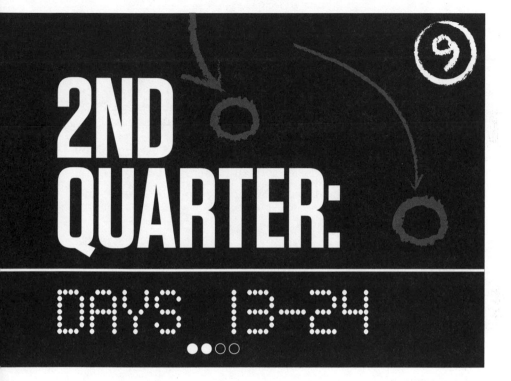

# 2ND QUARTER:

## DAYS 13-24

●●○○

OKAY, THE EXCITEMENT AND ADRENALINE FROM THE FIRST
QUARTER HAVE LIKELY DIALED BACK A LITTLE, BUT THE FIRE IS
STILL BURNING. It's time to settle in, go the distance, and do the
hard work of a champion. Some of your opponents might start to
waver and lose interest, but not you. You're focused! You can smell
victory. It smells like . . . bacon!

On page 182, you'll find a schedule that shows your workouts for
each day in this 12-day quarter. A little later in the chapter, you'll see
your second-quarter meal plan and a shopping list that'll make it
easy to get all the groceries you need to follow the meal plan. Here
are this quarter's new workouts. Enjoy!

# 110 PERCENT

**Goal: Keep track of your time and complete the challenge as quickly as you can.**

**Equipment: Track, football, or soccer field or someplace else that's big enough to run at least 50 yards straight (do twice for 100 yards)**

Run 100 yards, then stop and perform the indicated exercise. Move to the next sequence. Rest as needed but remember you are timing yourself. Record the time it takes for you to complete three rounds.

100-yard run followed by 10 Pushups

100-yard run followed by 10 Squats

100-yard run followed by 10 Burpees

100-yard run followed by 10 Forward Lunges (each leg)

100-yard run followed by 10 Pushup-Position Reachbacks (each arm)

100-yard run followed by 10 Shoulder Taps (each arm)

## Myth Busters

### Stretching Is the Best Way to Warm Up before Working Out

Rubbish. Have you ever heard the phrase "Don't stretch a cold muscle"? If you're stretching without doing an actual "warmup," that's what you're doing, stretching a cold muscle.

Although static stretching is one of several methods of increasing flexibility, it isn't a good choice for a warmup for exercising, or any other physical activity or sport. According to the NSCA (National Strength and Conditioning Association), performing static stretching before taking part in dynamic activity and exercise can have a negative effect on performance.

A recent study done by the *Journal of Strength and Conditioning Research*

# RAMBO

**Goal: Complete four rounds in 20 minutes.**

**Equipment: Stopwatch or clock with second hand**

Perform all exercises in the sequence shown below. Do each move for 30 seconds, rest for 30 seconds, and then moved to the next exercise. Do the circuit a total of four times in 20 minutes.

Jumping Jacks

High Knees

Squat Jumps

Boxing (left jab, left jab, right uppercut)

Lateral Bounds

concluded that stretching before a workout can leave you feeling weaker and more unstable than without stretching. Why is this? Well, it isn't fully understood yet. However, experts believe static stretching lessens the muscles' ability to store energy.

So what should you do to warm up? A better choice would be dynamic stretches and movements like those beginning on page 47. A proper warmup should always include movements and activities that bring blood flow to the muscles and increase the heart rate, such as leg swings, walking high knees to chest, and arm circles. This is like killing two birds with one stone. You get your body loosened up and warmed up all at the same time.

## FUNCTIONAL STABILITY WORKOUT #2

●●○○

Do each of the exercises in the order listed below. Complete all sets before moving on to the next exercise. Rest as needed. For exercise photos and descriptions, see Chapter 5.

| EXERCISE | SETS / REPS |
|---|---|
| Crunch | 2 / 15 |
| Single-Leg Bridge | 2 / 10 (each leg; hold each rep for 5 seconds) |
| Single-Leg Drop | 2 / 10 (each leg) |
| Bird Dog | 2 / 10 (each side) |
| Plank | 3 / 1 (hold each for 20 seconds) |
| Squat with Arms Up | 3 / 8 |
| Seated Russian Twist | 3 / 15 (twisting left and right = 1 rep) |
| Single-Leg Romanian Deadlift | 3 / 8 (each leg) |

## RIVAL STRENGTH CHALLENGE

●●○○

# 20 MINUTES IN HELL

**Goal: Perform as many rounds as possible in 20 minutes.**

**Equipment: Stopwatch or clock with second hand**

After a warmup, run through this 20-minute circuit, moving directly to the next exercise once you've completed all reps of the previous move. Repeat the circuit after completing the squats. Rest as needed but remember that this challenge is timed.

5 Mountain Climbers

10 Pushups

15 Squats

# Get More Calories Cheat Sheet

The food in the basic Workout War Lean Out Plan is based on a 2,000-calorie daily diet. But if you are on the big and beefy side and you are very active, you may need to add calories to hit your ideal daily total. That's where this food and snack calorie guide comes in handy.

## 25 Calories

1 cup air-popped popcorn
1 small glass of tomato juice
1 sugar-free Jello pack
½ cup vegetable juice
½ cup cooked or 1 cup raw vegetables (broccoli, beets, carrots, cauliflower, celery, cucumber, onions, peppers, mushrooms, salad greens, spinach, squash, tomato, and zucchini)
12 pretzels

## 45 Calories

1 tablespoon salad dressing
1 tablespoon sour cream
⅛ avocado
10 peanuts
1 tablespoon cream cheese
1 teaspoon light mayo
1 teaspoon margarine or oil
2 teaspoons peanut butter
2 tablespoons cream
6 almonds or mixed nuts
8 large black olives

## 50 Calories

1 cup air-popped popcorn with a handful of peanuts
1 cup grapes
1 handful of animal crackers
½ cup fruit cocktail
¼ cup reduced-fat cottage cheese

## 55 Calories

1½ oz low fat hot dog
1 oz lean beef or veal
1 oz lean ham or pork
1 oz lean lamb roast
1 oz luncheon meat
1 oz salmon or tuna
1 oz skinless chicken or turkey

## 60 Calories

1 cup fresh berries
1 cup fresh melon
1 small apple, banana, peach, or orange
⅛ melon
½ cup canned fruit
½ cup dried fruit
½ cup juice
½ grapefruit
17 grapes

## 75 Calories

1 egg
1 oz veal cutlet (unbreaded)
1 oz ground beef
1 oz low fat sausage
1 oz pork loin or chop
½ cup tofu

## 80 Calories

1 slice bread
⅓ cup cooked rice
½ cup cooked beans, peas, or corn
½ cup cooked cereal
½ cup cooked pasta
½ cup potato or sweet potato
½ English muffin
½ hotdog or hamburger bun
3 cups plain popcorn
¾ cup unsweetened ready-to-eat cereal
¾ oz pretzels
6" corn or flour tortilla

## 90 Calories

1 cup skim milk
2 slices of bacon
¾ cup nonfat yogurt
4 oz 2% low-fat small cured cottage cheese
Greek yogurt

## 100 Calories

⅓ cup Wasabi Peas
½ cup kale chips
¼ cup boiled Edamame with 1 tsp soy sauce (low sodium)
10 baked chips with ¼ cup salsa
1 oz smoked beef jerky—low sodium
2 tablespoons pumpkin seeds
40 Goldfish

# 2ND QUARTER WORKOUT SCHEDULE

●●○○

**Day 13:** Rival Strength Challenge: 110 Percent (page 178)

**Day 14:** Functional Stability Workout #2 (page 180)

**Day 15:** HIIT Workout: Rambo (page 179)

**Day 16:** Cardio

**Day 17:** Rival Strength Challenge: 20 Minutes in Hell (page 180)

**Day 18:** Functional Stability Workout #2

**Day 19:** HIIT Workout: Rambo

**Day 20:** Cardio

**Day 21:** Rival Strength Challenge: 110 Percent

**Day 22:** Functional Stability Workout #2

**Day 23:** HIIT Workout: Rambo

**Day 24:** Cardio

*Note:* You can do extra cardio every day, and as often as you would like. See the bonus cardio workouts beginning on page 203.

## LOG IT

Mark off each daily task as you complete it.

**WOD** = Workout of the day

**H₂O** = Drink 12 glasses of water

**MFP** = Logged on MyFitnessPal

| | DAY 13 | DAY 14 | DAY 15 | DAY 16 | DAY 17 | DAY 18 |
|---|---|---|---|---|---|---|
| | ☐WOD ☐H₂O ☐MFP | ☐WOD ☐H₂O ☐MFP | ☐WOD ☐H₂O ☐MFP | ☐WOD ☐H₂O ☐MFP | ☐WOD ☐H₂O ☐MFP | ☐WOD ☐H₂O ☐MFP |

| | DAY 19 | DAY 20 | DAY 21 | DAY 22 | DAY 23 | DAY 24 |
|---|---|---|---|---|---|---|
| | ☐WOD ☐H₂O ☐MFP | ☐WOD ☐H₂O ☐MFP | ☐WOD ☐H₂O ☐MFP | ☐WOD ☐H₂O ☐MFP | ☐WOD ☐H₂O ☐MFP | ☐WOD ☐H₂O ☐MFP |

(2ND QTR)

# (DAYS 13–24)

Here's everything you need to make the meals listed in this quarter's menu:

## PRODUCE

4 apples

3 fruits of choice
(1 cup or 1 piece = 1 fruit choice)

3 bananas

2½ cups grapes

1 carton berries of choice

3 cups cut mixed fruit

1 cup cut pineapple rings

1 lemon

1 lime

1 bag baby carrots

1 bag snap peas

1 bag fresh baby spinach

1 bag salad greens

1 bag shredded lettuce

1 bunch broccoli

1 bunch broccolini

3 large sweet potatoes

8 cloves garlic
(or purchased jar of minced garlic)

1 piece fresh ginger

1 bunch fresh cilantro

1 red or green bell pepper

2 green bell peppers

1 large bag mini bell peppers

3 medium yellow onions

1 large Idaho potato

1 bag celery sticks

1 small head lettuce

1 large zucchini

1 plum tomato

## DELI

3 ounces reduced-sodium turkey lunch meat

1 package turkey bacon

1 rotisserie chicken

## BAKERY

1 package whole wheat pita pockets

1 package Mission Carb Balance tortillas

1 package whole wheat hamburger buns

1 package whole wheat hot dog buns (like Healthy Life)

1 loaf whole wheat bread (like Nature's Own)

1 loaf French bread (whole wheat if possible)

## MEAT

3 pounds chicken breasts

4 boneless pork chops (4 ounces each)

4 pounds boneless beef tips

1 pound ground turkey

# WORKOUT WAR MVP

# AUSTIN GARCIA

| | | | |
|---|---|---|---|
| **AGE:** | 27 | **% WEIGHT LOSS:** | 9.30% |
| **OCCUPATION:** | Chef | **% BODY FAT LOST:** | 6.5% |
| **STARTING WEIGHT:** | 208.4 | **FAT MASS LOST:** | –16.6% |
| **ENDING WEIGHT:** | 189.0 | **LEAN MASS GAINED:** | + 2.8 pounds |
| **ACTUAL LBS LOST:** | 19.4 | **COMBO % LOST:** | 15.8% |

## Game Recap

This wasn't just a competition for Austin. It was a life changer. At 23, Austin felt a tightness and pain in his chest, classic symptoms of an impending heart attack. "It was one of the scariest moments, if not the scariest moment, in my life because my kids were in the car with me," he says. Fortunately, the scare sent him to seek medical help. Doctors warned that if he didn't lose weight and lower his cholesterol levels, he would be headed down the path to serious health complications, or even death within 2 years.

Austin credits the Workout War program with giving him the head start he needed to get back on track. "I wanted something that would motivate me, but also that I'd be able to do at home and wouldn't take me away from spending time with my daughters." The constant changes and new challenges of the workouts kept him inspired as the results started to show. "Now, I can actually see muscles in my body," he says. "I feel great, I have a ton more energy—every morning I want to wake up and do something."

## DAIRY

18 eggs

3 cartons pasteurized egg whites

1 package reduced-fat cheese slices

6 cups (6 ounces each) 0% Greek yogurt of choice + 2 cups (6 ounces) vanilla 0% Greek yogurt

1 package 100-calorie Greek yogurt cups

1 gallon 1% sweet acidophilus or fat-free milk

1 container feta cheese crumbles

1 bag reduced-fat Italian shredded cheese blend

1 bag reduced-fat Cheddar shredded cheese blend

1 package grated Parmesan cheese

1 tub low-fat sour cream or fat-free plain Greek yogurt

1 tub low-fat cottage cheese

3 packages low-fat string cheese

1 box Laughing Cow Light Cheese Wedges (flavor of choice)

1 tub Smart Balance Light butter spread

## FROZEN GOODS

1 box glazed baby carrots

1 bag broccoli florets

1 bag green beans

1 bag Green Giant Steamers Roasted Red Potatoes, Green Beans, and Rosemary Butter Sauce

1 bag Ore-Ida Steam n' Mash Cut Russet Potatoes

1 container (1.33 cups) frozen Birds Eye Steamfresh Lightly Sauced Creamed Spinach

2 bags Asian stir-fry vegetable medley, such as carrots, broccoli, and snow peas

2 bags frozen berries of choice

1 box Kashi Blueberry Waffles

1 bag cooked meatballs

## SHELF GOODS

1 can garbanzo beans (or chickpeas)

2 cans diced tomatoes

1 box 100-calorie microwave popcorn bags

3 packages Minute Brown and Wild Rice cups

1 box Kashi Chewy Granola Bars

1 box old-fashioned oats (or 1 box Quaker Weight Control Instant Oatmeal)

1 box original Cheerios

1 bag Bob's Red Mill Muesli

1 bag sliced almonds

1 bag whole almonds

1 jar natural jam (like Polaner)

1 bottle honey

1 jar nut butter (like Peter Pan Reduced Fat Peanut Butter)

1 jar Jif Whipped Peanut Butter

1 jar roasted red peppers

1 box Imagine or Pacific soup

1 box whole wheat stuffing mix

1 box whole wheat spaghetti (like Ronzoni Healthy Harvest)

1 jar reduced-fat olive oil mayonnaise

1 bottle Dijon or spicy mustard

1 bottle chili-garlic sauce

2 jars marinara sauce (like Ragú Light)

1 jar Classico Traditional Basil Pesto

1 bottle Buffalo sauce

1 jar tomato salsa

1 jar salsa verde

1 bottle horseradish sauce

1 bottle ketchup

1 bottle low-fat salad dressing
(such as Newman's Own Lite Low-Fat
Sesame Ginger Dressing)

1 can (6½ ounces) tuna, packed in
water

1 foil pouch (2.6 ounces) tuna,
packed in water

1 container whole grain Italian
seasoned bread crumbs (panko-style
optional)

1 box sweetener packets
(if desired, like Splenda or Truvia)

Jerk seasoning

Cayenne pepper

Dried parsley

Salt

Garlic powder

Ground cinnamon

1 bag all-purpose flour

1 bag coconut flour

Vanilla extract

1 bag dark mini chocolate chips

1 bottle extra-virgin olive oil

1 can nonstick cooking spray

1 box sugar-free hot chocolate mix

Make your life easier.
Stock up on
frozen vegetables

**Bold** denotes a recipe provided (see Chapter 7).

*Note:* If you have leftovers and do not see them on the menu in the following 4 days, freeze them for ease and convenience at a later date.

## Day 13

### BREAKFAST

1 serving **French Toast** (page 111)

1 tablespoon honey or pure maple syrup

1 cup berries or 1 banana on French toast

1 whole egg, cooked to choice, or 3 egg whites

### LUNCH

1 **Meatball Sandwich** (page 114)

1 container (1.33 cups) frozen Birds Eye Steamfresh Lightly Sauced Creamed Spinach

### SNACK

1 serving **Buffalo Chicken and Potato Wedges** (page 139)

### DINNER

2½ cups stir-fried vegetable medley (frozen, then stir-fry in 2 tablespoons Newman's Own Lite Low-Fat Sesame Ginger Dressing)

6 ounces chicken breast

1 cup Minute Brown and Wild Rice

### SNACK

8 ounces sugar-free hot chocolate made with 8 ounces fat-free milk

## Day 14

### BREAKFAST

5 egg whites (omelet)

1 cup broccoli

1 plum tomato, diced

¼ cup reduced-fat shredded cheese blend

2 slices whole wheat toast with 1 tablespoon natural jam

### LUNCH

2 servings **Buffalo Chicken and Potato Wedges** (page 139)

1½ cups steamed broccolini

### SNACK

4 **Mini Poppers** (page 140)

1 bag 100-calorie microwave popcorn

### DINNER

1½ cups whole wheat spaghetti (dry noodles with the diameter of a quarter)

¾ cup marinara sauce

3 frozen cooked meatballs

3 cups salad greens

2 tablespoons low-fat salad dressing

2 tablespoons reduced-fat shredded cheese blend

### SNACK

1 cup Cheerios

8 ounces fat-free milk

# Day 15

## BREAKFAST

1 smoothie

(blend 1½ cups frozen berries, 1 banana, 6-ounce cup 0% Greek yogurt, 8 ounces fat-free milk)

## LUNCH

1 Mission Carb Balance tortilla

1 tablespoon Classico Traditional Basil Pesto

2 ounces rotisserie chicken breast

2 tablespoons feta cheese crumbles

¼ cup roasted red pepper, cut into strips

1 cup fresh baby spinach

(roll above items up and wrap tightly in plastic wrap the night before and it will remain a nice, neat, tight roll!)

1 cup grapes

15 whole almonds

## SNACK

4 **Mini Poppers** (page 140)

1 bag 100-calorie microwave popcorn

## DINNER

2 servings **Chicken Fajitas** (page 130)

## SNACK

4 **Peanut Butter Balls** (page 136)

# Day 16

## BREAKFAST

1 breakfast sandwich (2 slices whole wheat toast, 3 cooked egg whites, 1 slice reduced-fat cheese, 1 slice turkey bacon)

1 fruit choice

(or you can substitute 2 Vitalicious Vita-Egg breakfast sandwiches + 1 fruit choice)

## LUNCH

2 **Tuna Pita Sandwiches** (page 112)

1 apple

1 Kashi Chewy Granola Bar

## SNACK

15 baby carrots

15 snap peas

¼ cup **Hummus** (page 144)

## DINNER

2 servings **Chicken Fajitas** (page 120)

## SNACK

20 dark cocoa–dusted almonds

# Day 17

### BREAKFAST

1 smoothie

(blend 1½ cups frozen berries, 1 banana, 6-ounce cup 0% Greek yogurt, 8 ounces fat-free milk)

### LUNCH

1 Mission Carb Balance tortilla

1 tablespoon Classico Traditional Basil Pesto

2 ounces rotisserie chicken breast

2 tablespoons feta cheese crumbles

¼ cup roasted red pepper, cut into strips

1 cup fresh baby spinach

(roll above items up and wrap tightly in plastic wrap the night before and it will remain a nice, neat, tight roll!)

1 cup grapes

15 whole almonds

### SNACK

4 **Mini Poppers** (page 140)

1 bag 100-calorie microwave popcorn

### DINNER

1 **Grilled Pork Chop** (page 119) (salsa verde optional, can substitute 1 tablespoon horseradish and mustard mixed)

1½ cups cooked green beans

1½ cups cooked glazed baby carrots

1 cup Minute Brown and Wild Rice

### SNACK

8 ounces sugar-free hot chocolate made with 8 ounces fat-free milk

# Day 18

### BREAKFAST

1 breakfast sandwich (2 slices whole wheat toast, 3 cooked egg whites, 1 slice reduced-fat cheese, 1 slice turkey bacon)

1 fruit choice

(or you can substitute 2 Vitalicious Vita-Egg breakfast sandwiches + 1 fruit choice)

### LUNCH

2 **Tuna Pita Sandwiches** (page 112)

1 apple

1 Kashi Chewy Granola Bar

### SNACK

15 baby carrots

15 snap peas

¼ cup **Hummus** (page 144)

### DINNER

4 ounces cooked chicken breast

1 large baked sweet potato

1½ cups cooked broccoli

1 tablespoon Smart Balance Light butter spread or 1 Laughing Cow Light Cheese Wedge (on potato)

### SNACK

4 **Peanut Butter Balls** (page 136)

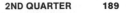

# LEGENDS:
## The Making of a Champion

# KARL MALONE
### aka "The Mailman"

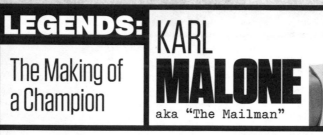

Karl Malone lived in the weight room and always went the extra mile during workouts. He loved to get a teammate or two involved in training with him, but only if they were 100 percent committed. He also liked to talk trash while working out or out on the court, but he always backed it up. That's why he was called "The Mailman"—because he always delivered. Karl loved to add variety to workouts during the off-season and take it outdoors; you could often find him running really big hills, or mountain biking, or chopping wood on his farm.

*"Every day, I try to do something a little bit harder than something I did the previous day. It could be something as small as lifting 5 pounds more, doing two more reps or going 0.1 mph faster on the treadmill. But I always find something to improve on from the previous workout. . . . There is just no substitute for hard work. I believe you get out of your body what you put into it."*

—KARL MALONE, on his workout ethic during his NBA days with the Utah Jazz

# Day 19

1 smoothie

(blend 1½ cups frozen berries, 1 banana, 6-ounce cup 0% Greek yogurt, 8 ounces fat-free milk)

**LUNCH**

2 cups Imagine or Pacific soup

1 slice whole wheat cheese toast
(1 slice reduced-fat cheese melted on bread)

**SNACK**

15 baby carrots

15 snap peas

¼ cup **Hummus** (144)

**DINNER**

2 cups **Easy Beef Stew** (127)

1 cup Minute Brown and Wild Rice

**SNACK**

4 **Peanut Butter Balls** (136)

# Day 20

**BREAKFAST**

2 Kashi Blueberry Waffles

1 cup berries

1 tablespoon honey or pure maple syrup

1 cup cooked egg whites

1 slice reduced-fat cheese in eggs

**LUNCH**

1 **Grilled Pork Chop** (page 119)
(salsa verde optional, can substitute
1 tablespoon horseradish and mustard mixed)

1 bag Green Giant Steamers Roasted Red Potatoes, Green Beans, and Rosemary Butter Sauce

**SNACK**

2 servings **Baked Zucchini Chips** (page 138)

½ cup marinara sauce

**DINNER**

2¼ cups **Asian Peanut Noodles** (page 128)

**SNACK**

1 bag 100-calorie microwave popcorn

4 tablespoons grated Parmesan cheese
+ black pepper (added to popcorn)

# Day 21

### BREAKFAST

5 egg whites (omelet)

1 cup baby spinach

¼ cup roasted red peppers, sliced

¼ cup feta cheese crumbles

1 toasted whole wheat pita bread with 1 tablespoon Smart Balance Light butter spread

### LUNCH

1½ cups **Easy Beef Stew** (page 127)

1 cup Minute Brown and Wild Rice

### SNACK

2 servings (4 pieces) **Mozzarella Sticks** (see page 141)

### DINNER

¾ cup **Easy Pulled Pork** (page 123)

1 whole wheat hamburger bun

2 servings **Baked Zucchini Chips** (see page 138)

¼ cup marinara sauce

### SNACK

4 **Peanut Butter Balls** (page 136)

# Day 22

### BREAKFAST

1 cup (6 ounces) 0% Greek yogurt

1½ cups mixed fruit

¼ cup Bob's Red Mill Muesli

1 slice whole wheat toast with 1 teaspoon Smart Balance Light butter spread

### LUNCH

1 large baked potato

1½ cups steamed broccoli

¼ cup low-fat shredded cheese

1 foil pouch water-packed tuna

### SNACK

2 servings (4 pieces) **Mozzarella Sticks** (page 141)

### DINNER

1 serving **Grilled Jerk Chicken** (page 123)

1 serving **Grilled Sweet Potatoes** (page 132)

1 cup steamed broccolini

1 cup grilled pineapple rings

### SNACK

4 **Peanut Butter Balls** (page 136)

# Don't Party Yourself out of the Running

As your trainer, I'm telling you, "Do NOT partake in alcoholic consumption if you're in this game to win!"

Look, I'm not clueless. I know there will be times when you come home from work and just really need to unwind after a tough day. You'll want to tune out the kids with the sound of a popping cap.

There will be times when you'll meet up with friend to watch the game and you'll find yourself lusting after an ice-cold beer like it's a Swedish swimsuit model.

I get it: You're human. So just in case you wuss out and decide to drink, I've put together this chart on the following pages so you'll know what you're getting yourself into. Alcoholic beverages, although tasty, are full of empty calories. Keep your cool and drink in moderation. In the immortal words of Ricky Bobby, Will Ferrell's character in *Talladega Nights*: "If you ain't first, you're last."

Don't drink yourself out of the ballgame, champ. Here's some advice from this bartender:

1. Preplan. What are you going to drink, and how many? Take a look at your eating and exercise log before going out for drinks. How many calories do you have in your expense account that you can allocate to a drink or two?

2. Once you've hit your predetermined number of drinks, stop drinking!

3. Chug a full bottle of water before you get to your watering hole.

4. Savor the flavor. Sip your drink. Don't chug it down like you did in college.

5. Don't order shots! Sip your drinks.

6. Having vodka or whiskey? Have it neat or on the rocks with water. Avoid the high-calorie mixers.

7. If you are going to mix, use a lighter version of juice or a diet soda.

8. Drink water or sparkling water in between drinks.

*(continued on page 196)*

# BELLYING UP AT THE BAR CHART

Here's what alcoholic beverages will add to your bottom line.

| DRINK | CALORIES |
|---|---|
| **REGULAR BEERS** | |
| Anheuser-Busch Ice Pale Lager | 171 |
| Beck's | 135 |
| Guinness Extra Stout | 176 |
| Harpoon IPA | 170 |
| Heineken | 166 |
| Killian's Irish Red | 162 |
| Long Trail | 163 |
| Molson Ice | 160 |
| Pete's Wicked Ale | 172 |
| Samuel Adams Boston Lager | 180 |
| Sierra Nevada Pale Ale | 176 |
| Yuengling | 142 |
| **LIGHTER BEERS** | |
| Amstel Light | 95 |
| Anheuser-Busch Light Pale Lager | 95 |
| Beck's Premier Light | 63 |
| Budweiser Select 55 | 55 |
| Corona Light | 99 |
| Heineken Light | 99 |
| Michelob Ultra | 95 |
| Miller Light | 96 |
| Miller 64 | 64 |
| Natural Light | 95 |

| DRINK | CALORIES |
|---|---|
| **MALT BEVERAGES** | |
| Angry Orchard | 190 |
| Four Loko | 337 |
| Mike's Hard Lemonade | 235 |
| Smirnoff Ice | 241 |
| Woodchuck Amber | 200 |
| **GIN (PER 1 OUNCE)** | |
| Gordon's | 96 |
| Seagram's | 104 |
| Tanqueray | 116 |
| **RUM (PER 1 OUNCE)** | |
| Bacardi | 98 |
| Captain Morgan | 86 |
| Malibu | 81 |
| **TEQUILA (PER 1 OUNCE)** | |
| Don Julio | 96 |
| Jose Cuervo | 96 |
| Patrón | 98 |
| **WHISKEY (PER 1 OUNCE)** | |
| Jack Daniel's | 98 |
| Jim Beam | 100 |
| Maker's Mark | 110 |
| **VODKA (PER 1 OUNCE)** | |
| Absolut | 96 |
| Grey Goose | 98 |
| Smirnoff | 97 |

# Day 23

## BREAKFAST

¾ cup old-fashioned oats cooked in 1 cup milk + water

1 apple, chopped, added to oats

1 teaspoon Splenda + 1 teaspoon cinnamon

1 tablespoon sliced almonds

(or 2 packs Quaker Weight Control Instant Oatmeal + 1 fruit choice)

## LUNCH

2 slices whole wheat bread

3 ounces turkey lunch meat

2 teaspoons reduced-fat olive oil mayo or spicy mustard or 1 Laughing Cow Light Cheese Wedge spread on bread

1 slice reduced-fat cheese

1 fruit choice

1 cup 100-calorie Greek yogurt

## LUNCH

2 servings (4 pieces) **Mozzarella Sticks** (page 141)

## DINNER

2 slices **Ma . . . The Meat Loaf** (page 121)

1½ cups cooked green beans

1½ cups Ore-Ida Steam n' Mash Cut Russet Potatoes, prepared

1 tablespoon Smart Balance Light butter spread

## SNACK

1 cup Cheerios

8 ounces fat-free milk

# Day 24

## BREAKFAST

1 cup (6 ounces) 0% Greek yogurt

1½ cups mixed fruit

¼ cup Bob's Red Mill Muesli

1 slice whole wheat toast with 1 teaspoon Smart Balance Light butter spread

## LUNCH

2 slices **Ma . . . The Meat Loaf** (page 121)

1 cup Ore-Ida Steam n' Mash Cut Russet Potatoes, prepared

1½ cups cooked green beans

1 tablespoon Smart Balance Light butter spread

## SNACK

1 serving **Cottage Cheese Salad** (page 137)

## DINNER

2½ cups stir-fried vegetable medley (frozen, then stir-fry in 2 tablespoons Newman's Own Lite Low-Fat Sesame Ginger Dressing)

6 ounces chicken breast

1 cup Minute Brown and Wild Rice

## SNACK

1 serving **Cookie Dough Yogurt** (page 137)

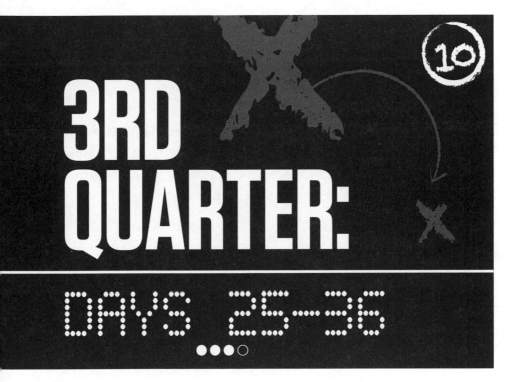

**NOW IS THE TIME THAT THE GAME CAN BE WON OR LOST—THE
CHOICE IS YOURS.** You need to pick up the intensity in your workouts
and stay focused on following your meal plans. The workouts should
be feeling harder. If not, kick it into gear and train like it might be
your last day. When your body or mind feel tired, tell them to "Shut
it!" Show no weakness! Keep your willpower all day, every day.

On page 202, you'll find a schedule that shows your workouts for
each day in this 12-day quarter. A little later in the chapter, you'll see
your third-quarter meal plan and a shopping list that'll make it easy
to get all the groceries you need to follow the meal plan. Here are this
quarter's new workouts. Enjoy!

## B-52 BOMBER

**Goal: Keep track of your time and complete the challenge as quickly as you can.**

**Equipment: Stopwatch or clock with second hand**

After an adequate warmup, start with walking lunges. Do 52 reps per leg, then move directly to burpees. Again, your goal is to do 52 quality reps for each exercise. Rest as needed, but remember your goal is to complete all reps in the circuit as quickly as possible.

| | |
|---|---|
| 52 Walking Lunges (each leg) | 52 Forward Lunges |
| 52 Burpees | 52 Jumping Jacks |
| 52 Squats | 52 Plank Pushups |
| 52 Pushups | |

*Are you tough enough for 52 burpees?*

## 99 PROBLEMS

**Goal: Complete the circuit as fast as humanly possible.**

**Equipment: Stopwatch or clock with second hand**

After warmup, do 99 body-weight lunges. Lunging with each leg equals one rep. (For mountain climbers, up and back with each leg equals one rep.) After completing 99 reps, move to the next exercise and so on. Rest as needed but remember that this is a timed workout. Try to complete the entire circuit as quickly as possible. Record your time and try to beat it the next time.

| | |
|---|---|
| 99 Forward Lunges | 99 Crunches |
| 99 Pushups | 99 Squats |
| 99 Jumping Jacks | 99 Mountain Climbers |

# BONUS DUMBBELL STRENGTH WORKOUT

**Goal: Complete 3 sets of 10 repetitions of each exercise.**

**Equipment: Dumbbells of various weights**

This bonus dumbbell workout may replace any of the Rival Strength Challenge in any of the quarters or the OT period, but wait until the third quarter when your body is ready for it. Don't do two Dumbbell Workouts consecutively. If you do the dumbbell program in place of the Rival Strength Challenge on the fifth day of the quarter, make sure you do a Rival Challenge on day 9.

Warm up first. Then, starting with Group A, perform each exercise in order for 10 reps per exercise. Rest for 90 seconds after completing all four exercises, then repeat the Group A circuit twice more. After the third round, move on to the Group B exercises. Perform 10 reps of each exercise and rest 90 seconds between each of the three rounds.

**GROUP A**

Goblet Squat

Standing Military Press

Romanian Deadlift

Biceps Curl

**GROUP B**

Squat & Press

Row

Chest Fly

Triceps Extension

# FUNCTIONAL STABILITY WORKOUT #3

●●●○

Do each of the exercises in the order listed below. Rest as needed. For exercise photos and descriptions, see Chapter 5.

| EXERCISE | SETS / REPS |
|---|---|
| Crunch | 2 / 15 |
| Single-Leg Bridge | 2 / 10 (each leg; hold each rep for 5 seconds) |
| Single-Leg Drop | 2 / 10 (each leg) |
| Bird Dog | 2 / 10 (each side) |
| Plank | 3 / 1 (hold each for 20 seconds) |
| Squat with Arms Up | 3 / 8 |
| Seated Russian Twists | 3 / 15 (twisting left and right = 1 rep) |
| Single-Leg Romanian Deadlift | 3 / 8 (each leg) |
| Inchworm, Hand Walkout | 3 / 6 |

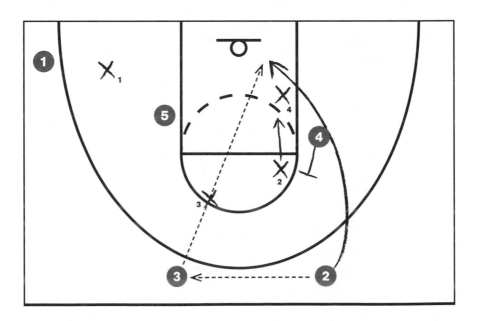

# THE PUNISHER

**Goal: Complete four rounds.**

**Equipment: Stopwatch or clock with second hand.**

Perform all exercises in the sequence shown below. Do each exercise for 40 seconds and rest for 20 seconds before moving on to the next exercise. Once finished with the last exercise, rest for 2 minutes before repeating the circuit.

Jump Rope

Squat Jumps

Lateral Bounds

180 Jumps

Burpees

## 8 Reasons to Drink More Water

1. Nearly 60 percent of your body weight is water.
2. Water makes up about 75 percent of your muscles' volume.
3. Even mild dehydration can cause fatigue and slow down your metabolism.
4. Proper hydration can increase your metabolism by 30 percent.
5. Drinking at least eight glasses of water per day can burn off almost 3,500 calories per year. That's 1 pound of weight loss. I want you to shoot for 12 glasses daily.
6. Water may help suppress your appetite.
7. Drinking enough water helps many ailments, including allergies, depression, digestive problems, chronic fatigue, constipation, urinary tract problems, and more.
8. Drinking enough water prevents water retention and improves muscle tone.

# 3RD QUARTER WORKOUT SCHEDULE

● ● ● ○

**Day 25:** Rival Strength Challenge: B-52 Bomber (page 198)

**Day 26:** Functional Stability Workout #3 (page 200)

**Day 27:** HIIT Workout: The Punisher (page 201)

**Day 28:** Cardio

**Day 29:** Rival Strength Challenge: 99 Problems (page 198)

**Day 30:** Functional Stability Workout #3

**Day 31:** HIIT Workout: The Punisher

**Day 32:** Cardio

**Day 33:** Rival Strength Challenge: B-52 Bomber

**Day 34:** Functional Stability Workout #3

**Day 35:** HIIT Workout: The Punisher

**Day 36:** Cardio

*Note:* You can do extra cardio every day, and as often as you would like. See the bonus workouts beginning on the next page.

## LOG IT

Mark off each daily task as you complete it.

**WOD** = Workout of the day

**H$_2$0** = Drink 12 glasses of water

**MFP** = Logged on MyFitnessPal

| WEEK 3 | DAY 25 | DAY 26 | DAY 27 | DAY 28 | DAY 29 | DAY 30 |
|---|---|---|---|---|---|---|
| | ☐WOD ☐H$_2$0 ☐MFP | ☐WOD ☐H$_2$0 ☐MFP | ☐WOD ☐H$_2$0 ☐MFP | ☐WOD ☐H$_2$0 ☐MFP | ☐WOD ☐H$_2$0 ☐MFP | ☐WOD ☐H$_2$0 ☐MFP |

| | DAY 31 | DAY 32 | DAY 33 | DAY 34 | DAY 35 | DAY 36 |
|---|---|---|---|---|---|---|
| | ☐WOD ☐H$_2$0 ☐MFP | ☐WOD ☐H$_2$0 ☐MFP | ☐WOD ☐H$_2$0 ☐MFP | ☐WOD ☐H$_2$0 ☐MFP | ☐WOD ☐H$_2$0 ☐MFP | ☐WOD ☐H$_2$0 ☐MFP |

# DOUBLE-DOWN BONUS CARDIO WORKOUTS

●●●○

Had enough? 'Course not, not if you want to win. Below are extra-credit workouts meant to give you an added cardio burn in your day or week. Some of these workouts will require equipment or a trip to a health club or gym.

## RUN, FORREST, RUN!

It's cardio time, so suck it up, Geneveve! Jump on a treadmill, find a track, or take it outside in front of your house. Lace up your running shoes and slap on a watch or something to keep time with.

Warmup: Walk or jog slowly for 5 minutes.

Hard: Run for 2 minutes at an exertion level between 6 and 8 on the RPE scale.

Easy: Run for 1 minute at an exertion level of 3 to 5.

Hard: 4 minutes

Easy: 2 minutes

Hard: 6 minutes

Easy: 3 minutes

Hard: 4 minutes

Easy: 2 minutes

Hard: 2 minutes

Easy: 1 minute

Cool down and stretch

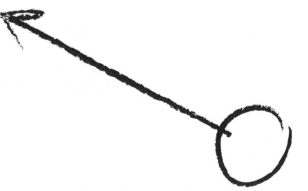

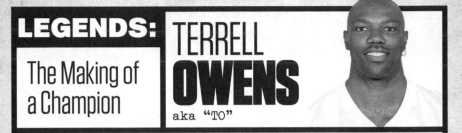

# LEGENDS:

## The Making of a Champion

# TERRELL
# OWENS

aka "TO"

We can all learn from the way T.O. approached training for football. He was always testing new workouts to find the most innovative and effective methods for getting stronger. He saw how training changed his body and performance when he was in college, and he carried that dedication to training right into his long pro career.

T.O. probably had one of the best performances I've ever seen coming off an injury and playing in Super Bowl XXXIX against the New England Patriots. Just 7 weeks earlier, the Philadelphia Eagles wide receiver broke his leg and tore a critical ligament in his right ankle. No one, including his doctors and teammates, thought that he would be able to play in the Super Bowl. Even though the Eagles lost 24–20 to the Patriots, Terrell Owens ended up catching nine passes for 122 yards.

He attributed that performance to the training regimen he was on while recovering. He never missed a workout and would always eat right to optimize his recovery in between workouts.

## THE GRIDIRON

You'll need an open place to run—a school football field would be perfect. However, if you don't have one close by, any open parking lot will do where you can mark off 10-yard lines with cones.

- Stand at the goal line facing the sideline with your right side toward the field. Side shuffle to the 10-yard line.
- Turn your back to the field and backpedal to the 20-yard line.
- Turn toward the sideline so your left side faces toward the 30-yard line and side shuffle to the 30-yard line.
- Turn facing the 40-yard line and sprint to it.
- Side shuffle (facing right) to the 50-yard line.
- Turn and backpedal to the 40-yard line.
- Turn and side shuffle (facing left) to the 30-yard line.
- Sprint the last 30 yards to the goal line.

Rest for 1 to 2 minutes and repeat back down the field. Start with one round and work up to as many as you can do in 20 minutes.

## BIKE YOUR BUTT OFF

For this workout, you'll need a stationary bike and a clock or stopwatch. With warmup and cooldown, it will take you 45 minutes to complete. You will alternate between an easy spin and a hard hill climb. Use a tension scale from zero to 10: Zero means there is no tension on the gear and 10 means you can't turn the pedal over. On the easy spin you want to be at about a 4 or 5; on the hill climb you want to be at 7 or 8.

- Do a 10-minute warmup in an easy gear (tension).
- 5-minute easy spin
- 5-minute hill climb
- 5-minute easy spin
- 5-minute hill climb
- 5-minute easy spin
- 5-minute hill climb
- 5-minute easy gear cooldown (3 on the tension scale)

# WORKOUT WAR MVP

## GREG PRESLEY

| | | | |
|---|---|---|---|
| **AGE:** | 46 | **% WEIGHT LOSS:** | 0.59% |
| **OCCUPATION:** | Hotel hospitality manager | **% BODY FAT LOST:** | 4.2% |
| **STARTING WEIGHT:** | 169 | **FAT MASS LOST:** | −7.3 pounds |
| **ENDING WEIGHT:** | 168 | **LEAN MASS GAINED:** | +6.3 pounds |
| **ACTUAL LBS LOST:** | 24.8 | **COMBO % LOST:** | 4.79% |

## Game Recap

When Greg heard that I was putting together some sort of a contest and there was money on the line, he was in. "I love sports, football pools, March Madness brackets, etc., so this was right up my alley; I didn't even need to know the specifics," says Greg. "I didn't have much weight to lose, but I definitely wanted to tighten up and put on some muscle, and this was just the motivation that I needed."

Then Greg's wife spoke up. She wanted in. But no women were allowed in this particular bro-only game, so Greg challenged his wife to a side wager: Loser does the dishes for a month. The couple found the workouts challenging but simple to follow. "I could do them almost anywhere, as I travel a lot for my job," says Greg. By the end of the program, Greg was fitter than he had been in many years. But his wife "totally kicked my ass," he says. She lost 15 pounds and more than 6 percent body fat. "She looked hot, so even though I lost, I was still a winner."

# THE PHELPS

This workout requires a 25- or 50-meter pool for lap swimming. (Skip this workout if you're not a good swimmer; always swim with a buddy.) The amount of time this workout takes will be determined by your swimming ability and speed.

- 100- to 200-meter warmup swim (any stroke you choose)
- Ten 25s (or five 50s) all-out sprint, resting 30 seconds in between bouts
- 200-meter easy recovery pace
- Six 25s (or three 50s) sprint, resting 30 seconds between bouts
- 100-meter cooldown using any stroke you like

# HAMSTER WHEEL

You'll need a treadmill for this workout, and you'll be doing intervals. How hard and/or fast you go will greatly depend on your athletic/ running ability. If you are a nonrunner, you can sprint the hard sections and walk or completely rest during the easy sections. If you are in good cardiovascular shape and can handle running the entire time, you will run hard or sprint the hard sections and jog the easy sections at an easier pace.

- Hard: Run for 2 minutes at an exertion level of between 6 and 8 on the RPE scale.
- Easy: Run for 1 minute at an exertion level of 3 to 5.
- 5 minutes of walking or slow jog warmup
- Hard: 30 seconds
- Easy: 30 seconds
- Hard: 45 seconds
- Easy: 45 seconds
- Hard: 60 seconds
- Easy: 60 seconds
- Hard: 90 seconds

- Easy: 90 seconds
- Hard: 60 seconds
- Easy: 60 seconds
- Hard: 45 seconds
- Easy: 45 seconds
- Hard: 30 seconds
- Easy: 30 seconds

Repeat back through the sequence up to three times. Cool down for 10 minutes by walking or jogging.

## THE CONEHEADS

You'll need an open place to run that has a good flat surface and three cones, or some way to mark stopping and starting points. Depending on your current fitness level, start with one sequence through the following workout, doing it in the exact order as laid out. As your fitness improves, add additional rounds. Make sure to cool down and stretch after you conclude your round(s).

- Warm up with a 5-minute walk or jog.
- From the starting cone (#1), run up to cone #2.
- Shuffle right to cone #3.
- Shuffle left to cone #2.
- Jog backward to the starting cone (#1).
- Do 20 Jumping Jacks.
- Repeat the cone sequence.
- Perform 10 Pushups.
- Repeat the cone sequence.
- Do 5 Burpees.
- Repeat the cone sequence.
- Cool down or start over from the top.

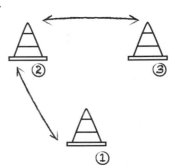

Place the cones 10 yards apart as shown below.

# (DAYS 25–36)

## PRODUCE

3 cartons berries of choice

1 Red Delicious apple +
4 apples of choice

2 fruits of choice
(1 cup or 1 piece = 1 fruit choice)

3 cups cut mixed fruit

3 cups melon cubes

4 cups grapes

2 lemons

1 lime

1 bag clementines

1 bag fresh baby spinach

1 bag salad greens

1 bag shredded lettuce

2 bags arugula

1 bag coleslaw mix
(shredded cabbage and carrots)

1 small head lettuce

1 bag broccoli slaw mix

1 bunch fresh cilantro

1 bag baby carrots

1 bag celery sticks

2 tomatoes

1 avocado

4 red bell peppers

1 orange bell pepper

2 medium green bell peppers

1 container cherry tomatoes

3 yellow onions

1 shallot

2 cloves garlic (or 1 jar minced garlic)

1 bag snow peas

3 bunches scallions

1 large sweet potato

2 large Idaho potatoes

4 Yukon Gold potatoes

1 tub guacamole

## DELI

1 package turkey bacon

1 rotisserie turkey breast

## BAKERY

1 package whole wheat pita pockets

1 loaf whole wheat bread
(like Nature's Own)

1 package Mission Carb Balance
tortillas

1 package small corn tortillas

## MEAT

4 pounds boneless beef tips

8 ounces seasoned pork tenderloin

2 chicken breasts

## DAIRY

18 eggs

3 cartons pasteurized egg whites

1 package reduced-fat cheese slices

1 cup (6 ounces) 0% plain Greek yogurt

1 cup (6 ounces) vanilla 0% Greek yogurt

1 cup Yoplait 100 Calorie Greek Yogurt

1 cup (6 ounces) 0% Greek yogurt of choice

1 cup 100-calorie Greek yogurt

1 gallon 1% sweet acidophilus or fat-free milk

1 bottle (8 ounces) low-fat buttermilk

1 bag reduced-fat Italian shredded cheese blend

1 bag reduced-fat Mexican shredded cheese blend

1 bag reduced-fat pepper jack shredded cheese

1 package low-fat string cheese

1 container feta cheese crumbles

1 tub low-fat cottage cheese

1 tub low-fat sour cream

1 tub Smart Balance Light butter spread

## FROZEN GOODS

1 box Kashi Blueberry Waffles

1 box Green Giant Baby Brussels Sprouts and Butter Sauce

1 bag Birds Eye Chopped Green Peppers and Onion

2 bags Birds Eye Recipe Ready Southwest Blend

1 bag Birds Eye Steamfresh Lightly Sauced Tuscan Vegetables with Marinara Sauce

1 bag chopped spinach

1 bag broccoli florets

1 bag haricots verts (fancy green beans)

1 bag (10 ounces) shelled edamame

1 bag (10 ounces) whole kernel corn

1 box Skinny Cow Ice Cream Sandwiches

1 box Vitalicious Vita-Top muffins or brownies

1 box Vitalicious Vita-Egg breakfast sandwiches (if not making your own)

1 pound (26–30 count) shrimp, cooked/peeled/deveined

## SHELF GOODS

1 bottle Dijon mustard or spicy mustard

1 jar reduced-fat olive oil mayonnaise

1 bottle low-fat salad dressing (such as Newman's Own Lite Low-Fat Sesame Ginger Dressing)

1 jar tomato salsa

1 jar jalepeños

1 jar dill pickles

1 can Italian diced tomatoes

3 cans plain diced tomatoes

1 can (8 ounces) artichoke hearts, packed in water

2 cans black beans

1 can (6 ounces) tomato paste

1 small can mandarin oranges, packed in juice

3 cans (7 ounces each) boneless, skinless wild Alaskan salmon

1 foil pouch (2.6 ounces) tuna, packed in water

1 can (6½ ounces) tuna, packed in water

1 box (32 ounces) reduced-sodium chicken broth

1 bag sliced almonds

1 box Kashi GO LEAN original cereal or 1 box Special K Protein cereal

1 bag Bob's Red Mill Muesli

1 box old-fashioned oats (or 1 box Quaker Weight Control Instant Oatmeal)

1 box Kashi Chewy Granola Bars

1 bag dark mini chocolate chips

1 bag dried cherries (just cherries, no added sugar or preservatives)

1 box raisins or currants

1 jar natural jam (like Polaner)

1 bottle honey

1 bottle pure maple syrup

1 box sweetener packets (if desired, like Splenda or Truvia)

1 box sugar-free hot chocolate mix

1 bag whole wheat orzo pasta

1 box whole wheat spaghetti (like Ronzoni Healthy Harvest)

3 packages Minute Brown and Wild Rice cups

1 box whole wheat couscous

1 box 100-calorie microwave popcorn bags

1 jar nut butter (like Peter Pan Reduced Fat Peanut Butter)

Vanilla extract

Salt

Garlic powder

Dried thyme

Cumin powder

Chili powder

Curry powder

Ground black pepper

Ground cinnamon

1 bottle apple cider vinegar

1 bottle rice vinegar

1 bottle extra-virgin olive oil

1 bag baked blue corn tortilla chips

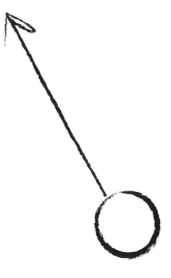

**Bold** denotes a recipe provided (see Chapter 7).

*Note:* If you have leftovers and do not see them on the menu in the following 4 days, freeze them for ease and convenience at a later date.

## Day 25

### BREAKFAST

¾ cup old-fashioned oats cooked in 1 cup milk + water

1 apple, chopped, added to oats

1 teaspoon Splenda + 1 teaspoon cinnamon

1 tablespoon sliced almonds

(or 2 packs Quaker Weight Control Instant Oatmeal + 1 fruit choice)

### LUNCH

2 slices whole wheat bread

3 ounces turkey lunch meat

2 teaspoons reduced-fat olive oil mayo or spicy mustard or 1 Laughing Cow Light Cheese Wedge spread on bread

1 slice reduced-fat cheese

1 fruit choice

1 cup 100-calorie Greek yogurt

### SNACK

1 bag 100-calorie microwave popcorn

2 pieces low-fat string cheese

### DINNER

2 cups **Shrimp and Edamame** (page 130)

1 cup whole wheat couscous

### SNACK

1 Skinny Cow Ice Cream Sandwich

## Day 26

### BREAKFAST

1 cup (6 ounces) 0% Greek yogurt cup

1½ cups mixed fruit

¼ cup Bob's Red Mill Muesli

1 slice whole wheat toast with 1 teaspoon Smart Balance Light butter spread

### LUNCH

1½ cups **Shrimp and Edamame** (page 130)

1 cup Minute Brown and Wild Rice

### SNACK

1 serving **Cottage Cheese Salad** (page 137)

### DINNER

1 **Taco Salad** (see page 115)

### SNACK

1 serving **Cookie Dough Yogurt** (page 137)

# Day 27

**BREAKFAST**

1 **Breakfast Burrito** (page 109)

1½ cups mixed fruit

**LUNCH**

2 cups **Spicy Vegetarian Chili**
(page 129)

¼ cup reduced-fat shredded cheese blend

**SNACK**

¼ cup **Spicy Artichoke Dip**
(page 143)

10 baby carrots

5 blue corn tortilla chips

**DINNER**

1½ servings **Fish and Chips Salad**
(page 122)

1 slice whole wheat bread

1 tablespoon Smart Balance Light butter
spread

**SNACK**

1 Vitalicious Vita-Top muffin or brownie

10 ounces fat-free milk

# Day 28

**BREAKFAST**

2 Kashi Blueberry Waffles

1 cup berries

1 tablespoon honey or pure maple syrup

1 cup cooked egg whites

1 slice reduced-fat cheese, in eggs

**LUNCH**

1 large baked potato

1 cup fresh baby spinach

½ cup **Spicy Artichoke Dip**
(page 143)

3 ounces rotisserie turkey breast

(stuff above in baked potato)

**SNACK**

3 **Curry Deviled Eggs** (page 145)

1 bag 100-calorie microwave popcorn

**DINNER**

4 ounces rotisserie turkey breast

1 cup whole wheat couscous

1½ cups Birds Eye Steamfresh Lightly Sauced
Tuscan Vegetables with Marinara Sauce

**SNACK**

8 ounces sugar-free hot chocolate made with
8 ounces fat-free milk

# Day 29

## BREAKFAST
1 **Breakfast Burrito** (page 109)

1½ cups melon cubes

## LUNCH
1 Mission Carb Balance tortilla

1 slice turkey bacon

1 cup fresh baby spinach

2 ounces rotisserie turkey breast

1 slice reduced-fat cheese

1 tablespoon spicy mustard

(make wrap of above)

1 cup grapes

15 smoked almonds

## SNACK
¼ cup **Spicy Artichoke Dip** (page 143)

10 baby carrots

5 blue corn tortilla chips

## DINNER
3 cups **Spinach Orzo** (page 135)

## SNACK
1 Skinny Cow Ice Cream Sandwich

# Day 30

## BREAKFAST
1 **Breakfast Burrito** (page 109)

1½ cups melon cubes

## LUNCH
1 cup **Chicken Curry Salad** (page 113)

2 whole wheat pita pockets

1 cup chopped lettuce

1 cup red grapes

## SNACK
3 **Curry Deviled Eggs** (page 145)

12 almonds

## DINNER
4 ounces seasoned pork tenderloin, roasted

1 cup Minute Brown and Wild Rice

1 cup apple, chopped and cooked into rice

2 tablespoons currants or raisins, cooked into rice

1½ cups haricots verts

## SNACK
1 tablespoon dark mini chocolate chips

¼ cup dried cherries

# Day 31

**BREAKFAST**

2 cups Kashi GO LEAN original cereal

1 cup berries

1¼ cups fat-free milk

**LUNCH**

1 Mission Carb Balance tortilla

1 slice turkey bacon

1 cup fresh baby spinach

2 ounces rotisserie turkey breast

1 slice reduced-fat cheese

1 tablespoon spicy mustard

(make wrap of above)

1 cup grapes

15 smoked almonds

**SNACK**

3 **Curry Deviled Eggs** (page 145)

1 bag 100-calorie microwave popcorn

**DINNER**

3 **Fish and Bean Tostadas** (page 124)

1 tomato, sliced

**SNACK**

1 Skinny Cow Ice Cream Sandwich

# Day 32

**BREAKFAST**

2 cups Kashi GO LEAN original cereal

1 cup berries

1¼ cups fat-free milk

**LUNCH**

1 cup **Chicken Curry Salad** (page 113)

2 whole wheat pita pockets

1 cup chopped lettuce

1 cup red grapes

**SNACK**

30 almonds

**DINNER**

4 ounces seasoned pork tenderloin, roasted

1 large sweet potato, baked

1 box Green Giant Baby Brussels Sprouts and Butter Sauce

1 tablespoon Smart Balance Light butter spread

**SNACK**

8 ounces sugar-free hot chocolate made with 8 ounces fat-free milk

# Day 33

### BREAKFAST

2 cups Kashi GO LEAN original cereal

1 cup berries

1¼ cups fat-free milk

### LUNCH

1 large baked potato

1½ cups steamed broccoli

¼ cup reduced-fat shredded cheese blend

1 foil pouch water-packed tuna

(stuff broccoli, cheese, and tuna in potato)

### SNACK

1 bag 100-calorie microwave popcorn

3 clementines

### DINNER

2 cups **Easy Beef Stew** (page 127)

1 cup Minute Brown and Wild Rice

### SNACK

1 tablespoon dark mini chocolate chips

¼ cup dried cherries

# Day 34

### BREAKFAST

1 **Baked Breakfast Pepper**
(page 110)

2 slices whole wheat toast with 1 tablespoon natural jam

### LUNCH

1½ cups **Easy Beef Stew** (page 127)

1 cup Minute Brown and Wild Rice

(freeze remainder of stew, portioned into 2-cup servings for another week)

### SNACK

1 apple

1½ tablespoons nut butter

### DINNER

3 **Fish and Bean Tostadas**
(page 124)

1 tomato, sliced

### SNACK

1 Skinny Cow Ice Cream Sandwich

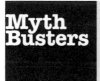

## Muscle Weighs More Than Fat

I would really love to meet the idiot who started this one. I can't believe how many people believe this and how many moronic trainers feed it to their clients. Think about it. You have two bags, one containing a pound of sand, the other a pound of rocks; don't they both still weigh a pound? Of course they do! A pound of anything is still just a pound.

So why do so many people believe muscle weighs more? Because muscle is about 20 percent denser than fat; thus, more of it can fit in the same size container.

Here's a visual. You've got two containers of equal size, and you filled one to the top with fat and the other with muscle. The one containing muscle would weigh more because more of it can fit into the container. The fat container weighs less because it's so thick, less of it can fit.

# Day 35

### BREAKFAST

1 **Baked Breakfast Pepper**
(page 110)

2 slices whole wheat toast with 1 tablespoon natural jam

### LUNCH

2 slices whole wheat bread

2 tablespoons nut butter

2 teaspoons honey

1½ cups grapes

### SNACK

1 bag 100-calorie microwave popcorn

3 clementines

### DINNER

6 ounces shrimp (cooked, peeled)

½ cup mandarin oranges

1 large red bell pepper, chopped (roasted if desired)

1 cup cooked whole wheat spaghetti

3 tablespoons low-fat salad dressing (such as Newman's Own Lite Low-Fat Sesame Ginger Dressing)

1 cup steamed snow peas

### SNACK

1 tablespoon mini dark chocolate chips

¼ cup dried cherries

# Day 36

### BREAKFAST

1 breakfast sandwich (2 slices whole wheat toast, 3 cooked egg whites, 1 slice reduced-fat cheese, 1 slice turkey bacon)

1 fruit choice

(or you can substitute 2 Vitalicious Vita-Egg breakfast sandwiches + 1 fruit choice)

### LUNCH

2 **Tuna Pita Sandwiches**
(page 112)

1 apple

1 Kashi Chewy Granola bar

### SNACK

30 almonds

### DINNER

6 ounces cooked chicken breast

1 cup cooked green beans + 1 cup cherry tomatoes, halved

¼ cup feta cheese crumbles, sprinkled over veggies

1 cup Minute Brown and Wild Rice

### SNACK

1 tablespoon dark mini chocolate chips

¼ cup dried cherries

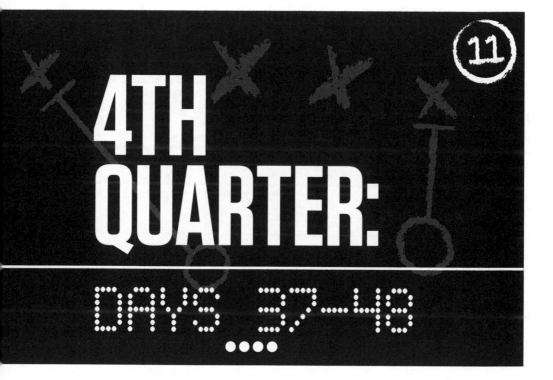

# 4TH QUARTER:
## DAYS 37–48

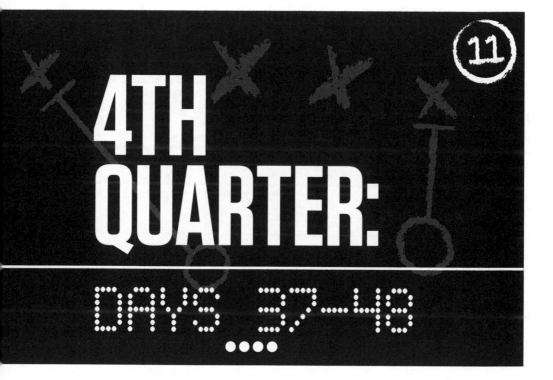

It's the fourth quarter, when the boys will be separated from the men. Now is the time to dig in. You've worked too hard to slack off now! Keep pushing and striving for greatness; focus on winning. See it. Smell it. Taste it. You are more dedicated than everyone else. They don't have the drive and willpower that you do. Keep taking it one day, one workout, and one meal at a time. Play like a champion.

On page 223, you'll find a schedule that shows your workouts for each day in this 12-day quarter. A little later in the chapter, you'll see your fourth-quarter meal plan and a shopping list that'll make it easy to get all the groceries you need to follow the meal plan. Here are this quarter's new workouts. Enjoy!

# DIRT OFF MY SHOULDERS

**Goal: Keep track of your time and complete the challenge as quickly as you can.**

**Equipment: Stopwatch or clock with second hand**

Begin with an adequate warmup and then start with shoulder taps. Do 20 quality reps, move on to the next exercise, and so on. Rest as needed, but remember your goal is to get through the circuit of five sets of shoulder taps and four sets of 100-rep exercises as quickly as possible.

20 Shoulder Taps

100 Squats

20 Shoulder Taps

100 Bicycle Crunches

20 Shoulder Taps

100 Walking Lunges

20 Shoulder Taps

100 Crunches

20 Shoulder Taps

*Hustle through these!*

# 21 JUMP STREET

**Goal: Complete three circuits of 21-rep exercises as quickly as possible while keeping track of your time.**

**Equipment: Stopwatch or clock with second hand**

After an adequate warmup, start the circuit of six jumping exercises. You'll do 21 reps of each. Once you complete the circuit, do it twice more for a total of three rounds. Rest as needed but remember that your goal is to complete the three rounds as quickly as possible. Record your time and try to beat it the next time you do this particular Rival Strength Challenge.

21 Squat Jumps

21 Jumping Jacks

21 180 Jumps (back and forth is one rep)

21 Side-to-Side Jumps (back and forth is one rep)

21 Lateral Bound (back and forth is one rep)

21 High Knees (both legs is one rep)

Repeat the circuit two more times.

# FUNCTIONAL STABILITY WORKOUT #4

●●●●

Do each of the exercises in the order listed below. Rest as needed. For exercise photos and descriptions, see Chapter 5. Complete all sets before moving on to the next exercise.

| EXERCISE | SETS / REPS |
|---|---|
| Crunch | 2 / 15 |
| Single-Leg Bridge | 2 / 10 (each leg; hold each rep for 5 seconds) |
| Single-Leg Drop | 2 / 10 (each leg) |
| Bird Dog | 2 / 10 (each side) |
| Plank | 3 / 1 (hold each for 20 seconds) |
| Squat with Arms Up | 3 / 8 |
| Seated Russian Twists | 3 / 15 (twisting left and right = 1 rep) |
| Single-Leg Romanian Deadlift | 3 / 8 (each leg) |
| Inchworm, Hand Walkout | 3 / 6 |
| Pushup Plank Matrix | 2 sets |

# BLACK OPS

**Goal: Complete four rounds in 20 minutes.**

**Equipment: Stopwatch or clock with second hand**

Perform all exercises in the sequence shown below. Perform each exercise for 45 seconds with *no* rest between exercises. Rest 2 minutes between rounds. Do four rounds.

- Jumping Jacks
- Mountain Climbers
- Jump Rope
- High Knees
- Side-to-Side Jumps

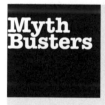

## Myth Busters

### Celebrities Have a Secret Technique for Losing Weight and Building Big Muscle

So we've all seen the celebrities in movies, magazines, and on TV who have had some sort of great body transformation. And we think, "Well yeah, I could do that if I had the money, a personal trainer, a private gym in my house, a massage therapist, cool workout clothes, and a beach to run on." Or you might think they did it by taking steroids, liposuction, some magic weight-loss pills, or lap band surgery.

Save your excuses! I believe the biggest reason why they can do it is not a secret trick, but money! They are *motivated* by money. Think about it—people like Jennifer Hudson, Charles Barkley, and Kirstie Alley all got paid millions of dollars to lose weight. Weight Watchers, NutriSystem, and every other weight-loss program out there pay their celebrity endorsers to lose weight.

Then there are the actors or actresses who get in great shape for a particular movie role. If Matthew McConaughey had a gut, women would not be lining up to go see his movies. Celebs have to look good or the money goes away. That's why they bust their asses in the gym and eat right every day. There's no magic pill. So remember their motivation is their *secret* advantage, and it can be yours, too.

# 4TH QUARTER WORKOUT SCHEDULE

●●●●

**Day 37:** Rival Strength Challenge: Dirt off My Shoulders (page 219)

**Day 38:** Functional Stability Workout #4 (page 221)

**Day 39:** HIIT Workout: Black Ops

**Day 40:** Cardio

**Day 41:** Rival Strength Challenge: 21 Jump Street (page 220)

**Day 42:** Functional Stability Workout #4

**Day 43:** HIIT Workout: Black Ops

**Day 44:** Cardio

**Day 45:** Rival Strength Challenge: Dirt off My Shoulders

**Day 46:** Functional Stability Workout #4

**Day 47:** HIIT Workout: Black Ops

**Day 48:** Cardio

*Note:* You can do extra cardio every day, and as often as you would like. See the bonus cardio workouts beginning on page 203.

## LOG IT

Mark off each daily task as you complete it.

**WOD** = Workout of the day

**H₂0** = Drink 12 glasses of water

**MFP** = Logged on MyFitnessPal

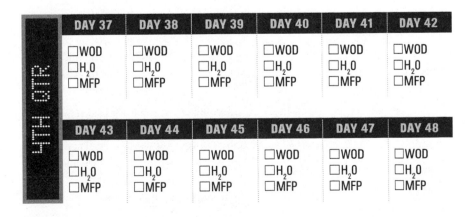

| | DAY 37 | DAY 38 | DAY 39 | DAY 40 | DAY 41 | DAY 42 |
|---|---|---|---|---|---|---|
| | ☐WOD ☐H₂0 ☐MFP | ☐WOD ☐H₂0 ☐MFP | ☐WOD ☐H₂0 ☐MFP | ☐WOD ☐H₂0 ☐MFP | ☐WOD ☐H₂0 ☐MFP | ☐WOD ☐H₂0 ☐MFP |
| | DAY 43 | DAY 44 | DAY 45 | DAY 46 | DAY 47 | DAY 48 |
| | ☐WOD ☐H₂0 ☐MFP | ☐WOD ☐H₂0 ☐MFP | ☐WOD ☐H₂0 ☐MFP | ☐WOD ☐H₂0 ☐MFP | ☐WOD ☐H₂0 ☐MFP | ☐WOD ☐H₂0 ☐MFP |

# 4TH QUARTER GROCERY SHOPPING LIST

●●●●

## (DAYS 37–48)

### PRODUCE

5 fruits of choice
(1 cup or 1 piece = 1 fruit choice)

7 apples

2 bananas

1½ cups melon cubes

3 cartons berries of choice

1 carton strawberries

1 cup grapes

3 lemons

1 lime

1 small head of lettuce

1 bag shredded lettuce

3 bags baby spinach

1 bag salad greens

1 bag coleslaw mix
(shredded cabbage and carrots)

1 bag baby carrots

1 bag snap peas

1 bunch broccolini

1 bunch asparagus

1 bag celery sticks

1 container cherry tomatoes

1 green bell pepper

1 red bell pepper

1 large bag mini bell peppers

3 Roma tomatoes

1 tomato

1 zucchini

1 bunch scallions

1 bunch cilantro

1 avocado

8 cloves garlic (or jar of minced garlic)

2 onions

1 spaghetti squash

5 medium sweet potatoes

8 small pieces sushi rolls (you should eat this within 2 days of purchasing it to ensure optimal freshness)

4 nigiri sushi (you should eat this within 2 days of purchasing it to ensure optimal freshness)

### DELI

6 ounces reduced-sodium turkey lunch meat

1 package turkey bacon

3 rotisserie chickens
(may want to wait and purchase one at the end of each week)

### BAKERY

1 loaf whole wheat bread
(like Nature's Own)

1 package Mission Carb Balance tortillas

1 package small corn tortillas

1 package whole wheat pita pockets

1 package whole wheat hamburger buns

1 package Flatout Light Original wraps

1 loaf French bread
(whole wheat if possible)

# A LEG UP

## Road Tripping without Tipping the Scale

At some point, you're going to need to travel either for work or vacation, both of which are invalid excuses for putting your competition on hold. Here's a list of helpful tips to keep you in the game, 'cause greatness doesn't take the day off.

1. **Pack snacks!** There are many quick and easy snacks you can put into a small bag or lunch box to nibble on while driving, or while sitting on the plane. If you pack the good stuff, you won't end up snacking on the salty, fatty prepackaged snacks at the airport.

2. **Stay hydrated.** Better to fill your belly with water than crappy fast food and gas station junk. Staying hydrated helps beat off feelings of hunger. (See "8 Reasons to Drink More Water," page 201).

3. **Choose healthy, calorie-friendly menu items.** Lucky for all of us, most restaurants now offer a few menu items for the health conscious. Even some fast-food chains like McDonald's are now putting the calorie content on their drive-up-window menus.

4. **Schedule your workouts.** Even if you're traveling for work, there has to be a 20-minute window somewhere in your day for a quick workout. The best way to make sure that you get it in is to make an appointment with yourself. Schedule it just like any other meeting.

5. **Don't make excuses.** Okay, so what if your hotel doesn't have a fitness center? You don't need one. You can work out in your room, in the parking lot, or at a local park. Rent a bike. Visit a YMCA. Pack hiking boots. Get creative. Don't make excuses; find solutions.

### MEAT

3 chicken breasts

4 tilapia fillets (4 ounces each)

2 pounds pork tenderloin

4 boneless pork chops (4 ounces each, center cut loin)

### DAIRY

18 eggs

3 cartons pasteurized egg whites

1 package reduced-fat cheese slices

2 cups (6 ounces each) 0% Greek yogurt of choice

2 cups vanilla 0% Greek yogurt

1 package 100-calorie Greek yogurt cups

1 gallon 1% sweet acidophilus or skim milk

1 bag reduced-fat Italian shredded cheese blend

1 bag reduced-fat Mexican shredded cheese blend

1 bag reduced-fat Cheddar shredded cheese

# WORKOUT WAR MVP

# DWIGHT MAUK

| | | | |
|---|---|---|---|
| **AGE:** | 32 | **% WEIGHT LOSS:** | 10.12% |
| **OCCUPATION:** | Chef | **% BODY FAT LOST:** | 3.6% |
| **STARTING WEIGHT:** | 409.0 | **FAT MASS LOST:** | −24.5 pounds |
| **ENDING WEIGHT:** | 367.6 | **LEAN MASS GAINED:** | +13.9 pounds |
| **ACTUAL LBS LOST:** | 41.4 | **COMBO % LOST:** | 13.72% |

## Game Recap

Dwight lost 41 pounds, but his biggest accomplishments were becoming more mindful of his calorie consumption (he's a chef, after all, surrounded by food to taste most of his working day) and using the functional workouts to get his body back into the swing of stretching and moving properly. "The Rival Challenges were great," he says. "They showed me how I could gain strength and lose weight in a short amount of time, which was very motivating."

Being able to do the workouts in the privacy of his home without weights or other equipment was a big plus. Dwight had no excuse not to work out, and when he finished the program, he gained the confidence to go back to the gym knowing he wouldn't feel out of place. "I learned how to move properly and push my body to its limits."

1 package grated low-fat Parmesan cheese

3 packages low-fat string cheese

1 box Laughing Cow Light Cheese Wedges

1 tub blue cheese crumbles

1 tub feta cheese crumbles

1 tub low-fat cottage cheese

1 tub low-fat sour cream

1 tub Smart Balance Light butter spread

1 bottle (8 ounces) orange juice

1 tub basil-garlic pesto sauce

1 package fresh Buitoni whole wheat cheese tortellini

## FROZEN GOODS

1 box Vitalicious Vita-Egg breakfast sandwiches (if not making your own)

1 box Vitalicious Vita-Top Corn Muffins

1 box Kashi Blueberry Waffles

1 bag green beans

1 box glazed baby carrots

1 box Brussels sprouts

2 boxes Green Giant seasoned veggies of choice

1 bag broccoli, cauliflower, and carrot medley

1 bag roasted red potatoes

1 bag frozen berries

1 bag Asian stir-fry vegetable medley, such as carrots, broccoli, and snow peas

1 bag Birds Eye Steamfresh Lightly Sauced Broccoli, Cauliflower, and Carrot with Cheese Sauce

1 bag Birds Eye Recipe Ready Southwest Blend

1 container Cool Whip Lite (or other brand 95% fat-free whipped topping)

1 California Pizza Kitchen Margherita Pizza

## SHELF GOODS

1 bottle Dijon mustard or spicy mustard

1 jar reduced-fat olive oil mayonnaise

1 bottle low-fat salad dressing (such as Newman's Own Lite Balsamic or Newman's Own Lite Low-Fat Sesame Ginger Dressing)

1 bottle horseradish sauce

1 bottle low-sodium soy sauce

1 bottle Buffalo sauce

1 bottle ketchup

1 jar jalepeños

1 bottle barbecue sauce

1 jar tomato salsa

1 jar salsa verde

1 jar dill pickles

1 jar kalamata olives, pitted and sliced

1 bag sliced almonds

1 bag mini dark chocolate chips

1 bottle honey

1 bottle vanilla

1 bottle ground cinnamon

1 bottle garlic powder

1 box sweetener packets (if desired, like Splenda or Truvia)

1 bag dried cherries

1 jar natural jam (like Polaner)

1 jar nut butter (like Peter Pan Reduced Fat Peanut Butter)

1 box old-fashioned oats (or 1 box Quaker Weight Control Instant Oatmeal)

1 box Kashi GO LEAN original cereal or 1 box Special K Protein cereal

1 bag sliced almonds

1 box Kashi Chewy Granola Bars

1 bag roasted almonds

Dried basil

1 bottle extra-virgin olive oil

1 can nonstick cooking spray

1 box seasoned bread crumbs

1 can spicy vegetarian chili

1 box tomato soup

1 can Italian stewed tomatoes

1 can navy beans

2 packages Minute Brown and Wild Rice cups

1 can (6.5 ounces) tuna, packed in water

1 can (7 ounces) boneless, skinless wild Alaskan salmon

1 large can (18 ounces) choice of boneless salmon or crabmeat

1 can garbanzo beans (or chickpeas)

1 can black beans

1 box Imagine or Pacific soup

1 box original Cheerios

1 box 100-calorie microwave popcorn bags

1 bag whole wheat orzo pasta

8 ounces diet root beer

1 tube prepared wasabi

1 box chocolate graham crackers

# 4TH QUARTER MEAL PLAN

●●●●

**Bold** denotes a recipe provided (see Chapter 7).

*Note:* If you have leftovers and do not see them on the menu in the following 4 days, freeze them for ease and convenience at a later date.

## Day 37

### BREAKFAST

¾ cup old-fashioned oats cooked in 1 cup milk + water

1 apple, chopped, added to oats

1 teaspoon Splenda + 1 teaspoon cinnamon

1 tablespoon sliced almonds

(or 2 packs Quaker Weight Control Instant Oatmeal + 1 fruit choice)

### LUNCH

2 slices whole wheat bread

3 ounces turkey lunch meat

2 teaspoons reduced-fat olive oil mayo or spicy mustard or 1 Laughing Cow Light Cheese Wedge spread on bread

1 slice low-fat cheese

1 fruit choice

1 cup 100-calorie Greek yogurt

### SNACK

1 Kashi Chewy Granola Bar

2 pieces low-fat string cheese

### DINNER

2 cups spicy vegetarian chili

2 Vitalicious Vita-Top Corn Muffins

¼ cup reduced-fat shredded cheese

### SNACK

1 cup Cheerios

8 ounces fat-free milk

## Day 38

### BREAKFAST

1 breakfast sandwich (2 slices whole wheat toast, 3 cooked egg whites, 1 slice reduced-fat cheese, 1 slice turkey bacon)

1 fruit choice

(or you can substitute 2 Vitalicious Vita-Egg breakfast sandwiches + 1 fruit choice)

### LUNCH

2 **Tuna Pita Sandwiches** (page 112)

1 apple

1 Kashi Chewy Granola bar

### SNACK

30 almonds

### DINNER

3 cups Asian stir-fry vegetable medley (frozen, then stir-fry in 2 tablespoons Newman's Own Lite Low-Fat Sesame Ginger Dressing)

4 ounces chicken breast

1 cup Minute Brown and Wild Rice

### SNACK

1 bag 100-calorie microwave popcorn

¼ cup grated low-fat Parmesan cheese

# Day 39

### BREAKFAST

¾ cup old-fashioned oats cooked in 1 cup milk + water

1 apple, chopped, added to oats

1 teaspoon Splenda + 1 teaspoon cinnamon

1 tablespoon sliced almonds

(or 2 packs Quaker Weight Control Instant Oatmeal + 1 fruit choice)

### LUNCH

2 slices whole wheat bread

3 ounces turkey lunch meat

2 teaspoons reduced-fat olive oil mayo or spicy mustard or 1 Laughing Cow Light Cheese Wedge spread on bread

1 slice low-fat cheese

1 fruit choice

1 cup 100-calorie Greek yogurt

### SNACK

1 Kashi Chewy Granola Bar

2 pieces low-fat string cheese

### DINNER

½ recipe **Mediterranean-Style Vegetables** (page 134)

1½ cups cooked spaghetti squash

1 tablespoon Smart Balance Light butter spread in squash

### SNACK

1 tablespoon mini dark chocolate chips

¼ cup dried cherries

# Day 40

### BREAKFAST

1 breakfast sandwich (2 slices whole wheat toast, 3 cooked egg whites, 1 slice reduced-fat cheese, 1 slice turkey bacon)

1 fruit choice

(or you can substitute 2 Vitalicious Vita-Egg breakfast sandwiches + 1 fruit choice)

### LUNCH

½ recipe **Mediterranean-Style Vegetables** (page 134)

1½ cups cooked spaghetti squash

1 slice whole wheat bread

1 tablespoon Smart Balance Light butter spread in squash

### SNACK

1 bag 100-calorie microwave popcorn

3 clementines

### DINNER

2 servings **Chicken Fajitas** (page 120)

### SNACK

1 cup Cheerios

8 ounces fat-free milk

# Day 41

**BREAKFAST**

2 Kashi Blueberry Waffles

1 cup berries

1 tablespoon honey or pure maple syrup

1 cup cooked egg whites

1 slice low-fat cheese, in eggs

**LUNCH**

¾ cup **Easy Pulled Pork** (page 123)

1 whole wheat hamburger bun

1½ cups frozen Birds Eye Steamfresh Lightly Sauced Broccoli, Cauliflower, and Carrot with Cheese Sauce

(should have pork and buns left over and frozen for this)

**SNACK**

6 **Mini Poppers** (page 140)

**DINNER**

4 nigiri sushi

4 spicy tuna rolls

4 California rolls

1 tablespoon low-sodium soy sauce

1 tablespoon wasabi

**SNACK**

1 bag 100-calorie microwave popcorn

¼ cup grated low-fat Parmesan cheese

# Day 42

**BREAKFAST**

1 **Breakfast Burrito** (page 109)

1½ cups melon cubes

**LUNCH**

2 cups tomato soup

1 whole wheat grilled cheese sandwich (1 slice low-fat cheese, ½ tablespoon Smart Balance Light butter spread on bread)

**SNACK**

6 **Mini Poppers** (page 140)

**DINNER**

1 serving **Greek Orzo Salad** (page 131)

3 ounces rotisserie chicken breast

**SNACK**

1 cup Cheerios

8 ounces fat-free milk

# Day 43

**BREAKFAST**

2 cups Kashi GO LEAN original cereal

1 cup berries

1¼ cups fat-free milk

**LUNCH**

3 ounces rotisserie chicken breast strips

4 cups fresh baby spinach

1½ cups sliced strawberries

3 tablespoons sliced almonds

3 tablespoons blue cheese crumbles

2 tablespoons low-fat salad dressing (like Newman's Own Lite Balsamic)

**SNACK**

1 serving **Cottage Cheese Salad** (page 137)

**DINNER**

1 **Grilled Pork Chop** (page 119) (salsa verde optional, can substitute 1 tablespoon horseradish and mustard mixed)

1½ cups **Sweet Potato Fries** (page 133)

1½ cups steamed broccolini

¼ cup ketchup or horseradish-mustard dipping sauce

**SNACK**

1 serving **Cookie Dough Yogurt** (page 137)

# Day 44

**BREAKFAST**

1 smoothie

(blend 1½ cups frozen berries, 1 banana, 6-ounce cup 0% Greek yogurt, 8 ounces fat-free milk)

**LUNCH**

1 Mission Carb Balance tortilla

2 tablespoons **Hummus** (page 144) or 1 Laughing Cow Light Cheese Wedge spread over the tortilla

3 ounces rotisserie chicken breast

1 cup fresh baby spinach or carrot/cabbage slaw

(roll this up and wrap tightly in plastic wrap the night before and it will remain a nice, neat, tight roll!)

1 box Green Giant seasoned veggies

12 roasted almonds

**SNACK**

15 baby carrots

15 snap peas

¼ cup **Hummus** (page 144)

**DINNER**

3 **Fish and Bean Tostadas** (page 124)

1 tomato, sliced

**SNACK**

2 **Chocolate Cloud Sandwiches** (page 142)

# Day 45

**BREAKFAST**

2 cups Kashi GO LEAN original cereal

1 cup berries

1¼ cups fat-free milk

**LUNCH**

1 Mission Carb Balance tortilla

2 tablespoons **Hummus** (page 144) or
1 Laughing Cow Light Cheese Wedge spread
over the tortilla

3 ounces rotisserie chicken breast

1 cup fresh baby spinach or carrot/cabbage
slaw

(roll this up and wrap tightly in plastic wrap
the night before and it will remain a nice, neat,
tight roll!)

1 box Green Giant seasoned veggies

12 roasted almonds

**SNACK**

1 serving **Cottage Cheese Salad**
(page 137)

**DINNER**

2 **Salmon Cakes** (page 119)

1 cup Brussels sprouts

1 cup glazed baby carrots

1 cup Minute Brown and Wild Rice

1 tablespoon horseradish sauce

**SNACK**

1 serving **Cookie Dough Yogurt**
(page 137)

# Day 46

**BREAKFAST**

1 smoothie

(blend 1½ cups frozen berries, 1 banana,
6-ounce cup 0% Greek yogurt, 8 ounces fat-
free milk)

**LUNCH**

2 cups Imagine or Pacific soup

1 slice whole wheat cheese toast (1 slice low-
fat cheese melted on bread)

**SNACK**

15 baby carrots

15 snap peas

¼ cup **Hummus** (page 144)

**DINNER**

1½ cups fresh Buitoni whole wheat cheese
tortellini

2 cups fresh baby spinach

1 tablespoon basil-garlic pesto sauce

1 tablespoon grated Parmesan cheese

**SNACK**

1 tablespoon mini dark chocolate chips

¼ cup dried cherries

# Day 47

**BREAKFAST**

2 cups Kashi GO LEAN original cereal

1 cup berries

1¼ cups fat-free milk

**LUNCH**

1 cup fresh Buitoni whole wheat cheese tortellini

2 cups fresh baby spinach

1 tablespoon basil-garlic pesto sauce

1 tablespoon grated Parmesan cheese

**SNACK**

1 apple

2 pieces low-fat string cheese

**DINNER**

⅓ frozen California Pizza Kitchen Margherita Pizza

4 cups side green salad

¼ cup dried fruit (in salad)

2 tablespoons nut pieces of choice (in salad)

2 tablespoons low-fat dressing of choice

**SNACK**

2 **Chocolate Cloud Sandwiches** (page 142)

# Day 48

**BREAKFAST**

1 serving **French Toast** (page 111)

1 tablespoon honey or pure maple syrup

1 cup berries or 1 banana on French toast

1 whole egg, cooked to choice, or 3 egg whites

**LUNCH**

⅓ frozen California Pizza Kitchen Margherita Pizza

4 cups side green salad

¼ cup reduced-fat shredded cheese in salad

2 tablespoons low-fat dressing of choice

**SNACK**

1 serving **Buffalo Chicken and Potato Wedges** (page 139)

**DINNER**

2 **Salmon Cakes** (page 119)

2 cups broccoli, cauliflower, and carrot medley

1 cup Minute Brown and Wild Rice

1 tablespoon horseradish sauce

**SNACK**

1 tablespoon mini dark chocolate chips

¼ cup dried cherries

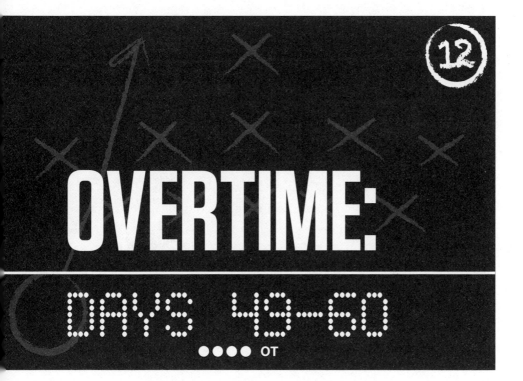

# OVERTIME:

## DAYS 49–60

●●●● OT

**WE'RE IN OVERTIME, BABY!** It's time to pull out all the stops. No cheating whatsoever! Turn up the workout intensity to epic levels; double up the cardio and workouts. Drink extra water and give each of the next 12 days hell. Finish this game knowing that you gave it everything you've got. Leave everything on the field so at the end of this, win or lose, you can walk away with no regrets or what-ifs. Let's get this thing done!

On page 243, you'll find a schedule that shows your workouts for each day in this 12-day period. A little later in the chapter, you'll see your overtime meal plan and a shopping list that'll make it easy to get all the groceries you need to follow the meal plan. Here are the OT's new workouts. Enjoy!

# 99 PROBLEMS

**Goal: Complete the circuit as fast as humanly possible.**

**Equipment: Stopwatch or clock with second hand**

After an adequate warmup, begin doing body-weight lunges. Do 99 total reps. Lunging with each leg equals one rep. (For mountain climbers, up and back with each leg equals one rep.) After completing 99 reps, move to the next exercise and so on. Rest as needed but remember that this is a timed workout. Try to complete the entire circuit as quickly as possible. Record your time and try to beat it the next time.

> 99 Forward Lunges
> 99 Pushups
> 99 Jumping Jacks
> 99 Crunches
> 99 Squats
> 99 Mountain Climbers

*You gotta problem with this?*

# 747

**Goal: Perform as many rounds as possible in 15 minutes.**

**Equipment: Stopwatch or clock with second hand**

Complete all the required reps before moving on to the next exercise. Focus on quality reps. When you finish with the last pushup, jump back into squats. Rest as needed but remember you are being timed.

7 Squats

4 Burpees

7 Pushups

*Note:* The exercise descriptions and photographs are found in Chapter 5.

## 6 Last-Minute Steps to Dominate Your Competition

You want to win, right? Well, now is not the time to fall back into your old habits. Now more than ever you need to put your nose to the grindstone and keep good habits going and then some. When you think you've given everything you've got—give more. Crush your comfort zone, take your body places you didn't know it could go. Remember that if you want something bad enough, you must break through short-term pain to achieve that long-term pleasure. Here are some final tips for the home stretch.

1. Drink more water! How much more? Until your eyes float.
2. Lower your salt intake. Don't salt your food; it causes fluid retention aka water weight.
3. Crank up the cardio. Think higher intensity and longer duration. Make your body beg for mercy.
4. Cut back your daily caloric intake by 200 to 500 calories, making sure not to go below 1,500 per day.
5. Do the Turbo Eating Plan (see page 103) for the last 7 days.
6. Go overboard. Think like a winner. Act like a winner.

# 20 MINUTES IN HELL

**Goal: Perform as many rounds as possible in 20 minutes.**

**Equipment: Stopwatch or clock with second hand**

After a warmup, run through this 20-minute circuit, moving directly to the next exercise once you've completed all reps of the previous move. Repeat the circuit after completing the squats. Rest as needed but remember that this challenge is timed.

> 5 Mountain Climbers
>
> 10 Pushups
>
> 15 Squats

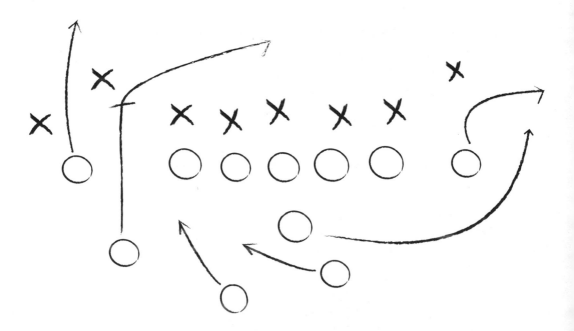

# DIRT OFF MY SHOULDERS

**Goal:** Keep track of your time and complete the challenge as quickly as you can.

**Equipment:** Stopwatch or clock with second hand

Begin with an adequate warmup, and then start with shoulder taps. Do 20 quality reps, move on to the next exercise, and so on. Rest as needed, but remember your goal is to get through the circuit of five sets of shoulder taps and four sets of 100-rep exercises as quickly as possible.

- 20 Shoulder Taps
- 100 Squats
- 20 Shoulder Taps
- 100 Bicycle Crunches
- 20 Shoulder Taps
- 100 Walking Lunges
- 20 Shoulder Taps
- 100 Crunches
- 20 Shoulder Taps

# 110 PERCENT

**Goal: Keep track of your time and complete the challenge as quickly as you can.**

**Equipment: Track, football, or soccer field or someplace else that's big enough to run at least 50 yards straight (do twice for 100 yards)**

Run 100 yards, then stop and perform the indicated exercise. Move to the next sequence. Rest as needed but remember you are timing yourself. Record the time it takes for you to complete three rounds.

100-yard run followed by 10 Pushups

100-yard run followed by 10 Squats

100-yard run followed by 10 Burpees

100-yard run followed by 10 Forward Lunges (each leg)

100-yard run followed by 10 Pushup-Position Reachbacks (each arm)

100-yard run followed by 10 Shoulder Taps (each arm)

# FUNCTIONAL STABILITY WORKOUT #5

●●●● OT

Do each of the exercises in the order listed below. Rest as needed. For exercise photos and descriptions, see Chapter 5. Complete all sets before moving on to the next exercise.

| EXERCISE | SETS / REPS |
|---|---|
| Crunch | 2 / 15 |
| Single-Leg Bridge | 2 / 10 (each leg; hold each rep for 5 seconds) |
| Single-Leg Drop | 2 / 10 (each leg) |
| Bird Dog | 2 / 10 (each side) |
| Plank | 3 / 1 (hold each for 20 seconds) |
| Squat with Arms Up | 3 / 8 |
| Seated Russian Twist | 3 / 15 (twisting right and left = 1 rep) |
| Single-Leg Romanian Deadlift | 3 / 8 (each leg) |
| Inchworm, Hand Walkup | 3 / 6 |
| Pushup Plank Matrix | 2 sets |
| Forward Lunge | 3 / 8 (each leg) |

# THE PUNISHER

**Goal: Complete four circuits.**

**Equipment: Stopwatch or clock with second hand**

Perform all exercises in the sequence shown below for 1 minute with NO rest between exercises. Rest for 1 minute after each round. Repeat three more times for a total of four rounds.

- Jump Rope
- Squat Jumps
- Lateral Bounds
- 180 Jumps
- Burpees

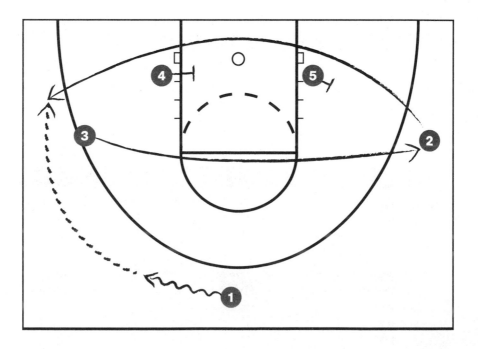

# YOUR OVERTIME WORKOUT SCHEDULE
●●●● OT

**Day 49:** Rival Strength Challenge: 99 Problems (page 236)

**Day 50:** Functional Stability Workout #5 (page 241)

**Day 51:** HIIT Workout: The Punisher (opposite page)

**Day 52:** Rival Strength Challenge: 747 (page 237)

**Day 53:** Rival Strength Challenge: 20 Minutes in Hell (page 238)

**Day 54:** Cardio

**Day 55:** HIIT Workout: The Punisher

**Day 56:** Rival Strength Challenge: Dirt off My Shoulders (page 239)

**Day 57:** Cardio

**Day 58:** Functional Stability Workout #5

**Day 59:** HIIT Workout: The Punisher

**Day 60:** Rival Strength Challenge: 110 Percent (page 240)

*Note:* You can do extra cardio every day, and as often as you would like. See the bonus cardio workouts beginning on page 205.

## LOG IT

Mark off each daily task as you complete it.

**WOD** = Workout of the day

$H_2O$ = Drink 12 glasses of water

**MFP** = Logged on MyFitnessPal

| | DAY 49 | DAY 50 | DAY 51 | DAY 52 | DAY 53 | DAY 54 |
|---|---|---|---|---|---|---|
| OVERTIME | ☐WOD ☐$H_2O$ ☐MFP | ☐WOD ☐$H_2O$ ☐MFP | ☐WOD ☐$H_2O$ ☐MFP | ☐WOD ☐$H_2O$ ☐MFP | ☐WOD ☐$H_2O$ ☐MFP | ☐WOD ☐$H_2O$ ☐MFP |
| | **DAY 55** | **DAY 56** | **DAY 57** | **DAY 58** | **DAY 59** | **DAY 60** |
| | ☐WOD ☐$H_2O$ ☐MFP | ☐WOD ☐$H_2O$ ☐MFP | ☐WOD ☐$H_2O$ ☐MFP | ☐WOD ☐$H_2O$ ☐MFP | ☐WOD ☐$H_2O$ ☐MFP | ☐WOD ☐$H_2O$ ☐MFP |

# (DAYS 49–60)

## PRODUCE

2 fruits of choice
(1 cup or 1 piece = 1 fruit choice)

7 apples + 1 Red Delicious apple
+ 1 green apple

4 bananas or 4 more apples

3 cartons berries of choice
+ 1 carton blueberries

2½ cups mixed melon cubes

4½ cups grapes

3 lemons

3 limes

1 bag clementines

1 bag celery sticks

1 bag baby carrots

1 bag snap peas

1 bag chopped or shredded lettuce

1 bag coleslaw mix
(shredded cabbage and carrots)

1 bag fresh baby spinach

1 bag salad greens

1 bag arugula

6 large red bell peppers

1 green bell pepper

1 zucchini

3 onions

1 bunch cilantro

1 carton cherry tomatoes

2 bunches broccolini

1 bunch asparagus

1 spaghetti squash

7 cloves garlic (or 1 jar minced garlic)

1 bunch scallions

4 Yukon Gold potatoes

3 pounds sweet potatoes

1 shallot

1 tub guacamole

8 small pieces sushi rolls (you should
eat this within 2 days of purchasing it
to ensure optimal freshness)

4 nigiri sushi (you should eat this
within 2 days of purchasing it to
ensure optimal freshness)

## DELI

3 ounces reduced-sodium turkey
lunch meat

1 package turkey bacon

1 rotisserie chicken

## BAKERY

1 loaf whole wheat bread
(like Nature's Own)

1 package whole wheat pita pockets

1 package whole wheat hot dog buns
(like Healthy Life)

1 loaf French bread
(whole wheat if possible)

1 package Mission Carb
Balance tortillas

## Crunches Will Give You a Six-Pack

All right, we all want the six-pack abs, and we think that doing more crunches, situps, planks, and leg raises will get us there. But in reality, what is holding us back from the six-pack is usually the six-packs of beer and the junk food we eat with it. Yes, that's right, it's your diet that gives you that layer of fat over your abdominal wall. Blame the beer, pizza, chips, cheeseburgers, and all the other junk food that is readily available.

For most of us guys, the first place on our bodies that starts to accumulate this excess fat is our stomachs. The beer belly, the 30-pack, the liquid grain storage facility, the spare tire, love handles, a Dunlap (the belly has "dun lapped" over your belt), the keg, the Buddha, the guzzle gut, beer muscles, the pooch, the Budweiser tumor, blubber belly . . . I could go on and on. The names we have given our fat stomachs are funny, but yet, Houston, we have a problem.

So here's the deal: If you want the six-pack abs, you've got to eat good, clean foods. Not once in a blue moon—all the time. You've got to stick with that if you want to see any ripples on the washboard.

Next, you've got to burn fat through exercise. Now when you do start burning off fat, it doesn't just come off the belly, it comes off the entire body, not just one area. You can't spot reduce and pick the area where you want the fat to come off. So you have to get your total body-fat percentage down if the six-pack is gonna come through.

With all that said, I do want you to do abdominal exercises (the crunches, planks, and more) because they are very important in making the body fit and healthy. But if you think that just doing the crunches every day, or using the amazing ab-sculpting machine you see in an infomercial every day, is going to get the job done, you are living in a dream. So remember, it takes a clean diet, exercise to burn fat, and abdominal exercises to strengthen your core to turn that gut into a six-pack.

# CARL SCHULTHEIS

| | | | |
|---|---|---|---|
| **AGE:** | 37 | **% WEIGHT LOSS:** | 4.29% |
| **OCCUPATION:** | Chef | **% BODY FAT LOST:** | 7.7% |
| **STARTING WEIGHT:** | 302.4 | **FAT MASS LOST:** | −26.1 pounds |
| **ENDING WEIGHT:** | 289.4 | **LEAN MASS GAINED:** | +13.1 pounds |
| **ACTUAL LBS LOST:** | 13 | **COMBO % LOST:** | 11.99% |

### Game Recap

Carl lost 26 pounds of fat and gained 13 pounds of lean muscle—something he would have never accomplished, he says, had it not been for the Workout War test panel contest. "The competition aspect makes losing weight more fun, and it drives you to push harder to meet your goals," he says.

The program delivered two key revelations that he says have become part of his lifestyle. One is drinking more water. "I realized how little water I was drinking every day and how much better I felt when I was better hydrated." Second: Using a calorie- and workout-tracking program is critical to staying the course. "Logging your food on MyFitnessPal forces you to realize true portion sizes and also recognize that weight loss is a daily challenge, that if you cheat one day, you are back to square one the next."

## MEAT

4 chicken breasts

5 ounces pork tenderloin

4 tilapia fillets (4 ounces each)

4 ounces salmon fillet

## DAIRY

18 eggs

3 cartons pasteurized egg whites

1 package reduced-fat cheese slices

1 cup (6 ounces) plain 0% Greek yogurt

1 cup (6 ounces) vanilla 0% Greek yogurt

1 package 100-calorie Greek yogurt cups

1 gallon 1% sweet acidophilus or fat-free milk

2 bags reduced-fat Italian shredded cheese blend

1 bag reduced-fat shredded Cheddar cheese blend

1 bag reduced-fat pepper jack shredded cheese

2 packages low-fat string cheese

1 tub feta cheese crumbles

1 bottle (8 ounces) orange juice

1 bottle (8 ounces) low-fat buttermilk

## FROZEN GOODS

1 box organic Vitalicious Vita-Egg breakfast sandwiches (if not making your own)

1 box Kashi Blueberry Waffles

1 bag roasted red potatoes

1 bag haricots verts (fancy green beans)

1 bag (10 ounces) shelled edamame

1 bag (10 ounces) corn kernels

1 bag chopped spinach

1 bag Birds Eye Steamfresh Lightly Sauced Creamed Spinach

1 bag Birds Eye Recipe Ready Southwest Blend

1 bag (1 pound, 26–30 count) cooked/peeled shrimp

1 bag cooked meatballs

1 container Cool Whip Lite (or other 95% fat-free whipped topping)

1 box Skinny Cow Ice Cream Sandwiches

1 box Vitalicious Vita-Top muffins or brownies

## SHELF GOODS

1 bottle Dijon mustard or spicy mustard

1 jar reduced-fat olive oil mayonnaise

1 bottle low-fat salad dressing

1 jar tomato salsa

1 bottle Buffalo sauce

1 tube prepared wasabi paste

1 bottle low-sodium soy sauce

2 jars marinara sauce (like Ragú Light)

1 jar (8 ounces) artichoke hearts, in water

1 can navy beans

2 cans black beans

1 can garbanzo beans (chickpeas)

1 can Italian stewed tomatoes

1 can diced Italian tomatoes

2 boxes reduced-sodium chicken broth

2 cans (7 ounces each) boneless, skinless wild Alaskan salmon

1 box whole wheat spaghetti (like Ronzoni Healthy Harvest)

1 bag whole wheat orzo pasta

1 bag brown rice

2 packages Minute Brown and Wild Rice cups

1 bag sliced almonds

1 bag almonds

1 bag mini dark chocolate chips

1 bottle honey

1 jar natural jam (like Polaner)

1 jar nut butter (like Peter Pan Reduced Fat Peanut Butter)

1 jar Jif Whipped Peanut Butter

1 bag coconut flour

Vanilla extract

Curry powder

Ground cumin

Ground cinnamon

Salt

Garlic powder

Dried basil

Dried thyme

1 bottle extra-virgin olive oil

1 bottle apple cider vinegar

1 bottle rice vinegar

1 box of sweetener packets (if desired, like Splenda or Truvia)

1 box golden raisins or currants

1 box old-fashioned oats (or 1 box Quaker Weight Control Instant Oatmeal if not making your own)

1 box original Cheerios

1 box 100-calorie microwave popcorn bags

1 box sugar-free hot chocolate mix

1 box chocolate graham crackers

1 bag baked blue corn tortilla chips

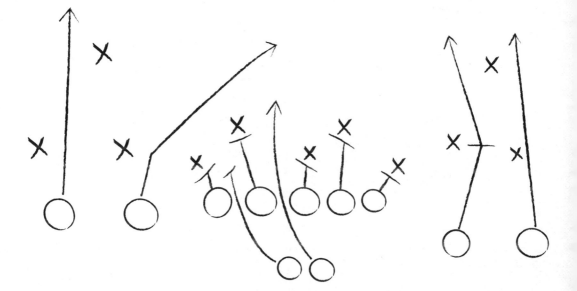

**Bold** denotes a recipe provided (see Chapter 7).

*Note:* If you have leftovers and do not see them on the menu in the following 4 days, freeze them for ease and convenience at a later date.

## Day 49

### BREAKFAST

1 serving **French Toast** (page 111)

1 tablespoon honey or pure maple syrup

1 cup berries or 1 banana on French toast

1 whole egg, cooked to choice, or 3 egg whites

### LUNCH

2 servings **Buffalo Chicken and Potato Wedges** (page 139)

1½ cups broccolini, steamed

### SNACK

15 baby carrots

15 snap peas

¼ cup **Hummus** (page 144)

### DINNER

4 ounces poached salmon

1½ cups asparagus

2 cups roasted new potatoes

2 tablespoons **Spicy Mustard Sauce** (page 135)

### SNACK

2 **Chocolate Cloud Sandwiches** (page 142)

## Day 50

### BREAKFAST

¾ cup old-fashioned oats cooked in 1 cup milk + water

1 apple, chopped, added to oats

1 teaspoon Splenda + 1 teaspoon cinnamon

1 tablespoon sliced almonds

(or 2 packs Quaker Weight Control Instant Oatmeal + 1 fruit choice)

### LUNCH

1 cup **Chicken Curry Salad** (page 113)

2 whole wheat pita pockets

1 cup chopped lettuce

1 cup red grapes

### SNACK

1 bag 100-calorie microwave popcorn

2 pieces low-fat string cheese

### DINNER

1 serving **Grilled Tilapia Fillet** (page 117)

½ recipe **Mediterranean-Style Vegetables** (page 134)

1½ cups cooked spaghetti squash

1 tablespoon Smart Balance Light butter spread in squash

### SNACK

4 **Peanut Butter Balls** (page 136)

# Day 51

### BREAKFAST

1 breakfast sandwich (2 slices whole wheat toast, 3 cooked egg whites, 1 slice reduced-fat cheese, 1 slice turkey bacon)

1 fruit choice

(or you can substitute 2 Vitalicious Vita-Egg breakfast sandwiches + 1 fruit choice)

### LUNCH

½ recipe **Mediterranean-Style Vegetables** (page 134)

1½ cups cooked spaghetti squash

1 slice whole wheat bread

1 tablespoon Smart Balance Light butter spread in squash

### SNACK

1 apple or banana

1½ tablespoons nut butter

### DINNER

5 ounces pork tenderloin, roasted

1 cup Minute Brown and Wild Rice

1 cup apple, chopped and cooked into wild rice

2 tablespoons currants or raisins, cooked into rice

1½ cups haricots verts

### SNACK

8 ounces sugar-free hot chocolate made with 8 ounces fat-free milk

# Day 52

### BREAKFAST

¾ cup old-fashioned oats cooked in 1 cup milk + water

1 apple, chopped, added to oats

1 teaspoon Splenda + 1 teaspoon cinnamon

1 tablespoon sliced almonds

(or 2 packs Quaker Weight Control Instant Oatmeal + 1 fruit choice)

### LUNCH

1 cup **Chicken Curry Salad** (page 113)

2 whole wheat pita pockets

1 cup chopped lettuce

1 cup red grapes

### SNACK

1 bag 100-calorie microwave popcorn

2 pieces low-fat string cheese

### DINNER

2 cups **Shrimp and Edamame** (page 130)

1 cup Minute Brown and Wild Rice

### SNACK

4 **Peanut Butter Balls** (page 136)

# Day 53

### BREAKFAST

1 breakfast sandwich (2 slices whole wheat toast, 3 cooked egg whites, 1 slice reduced-fat cheese, 1 slice turkey bacon)

1 fruit choice

(or you can substitute 2 Vitalicious Vita-Egg breakfast sandwiches + 1 fruit choice)

### LUNCH

1½ cups **Shrimp and Edamame** (page 130)

1 cup Minute Brown and Wild Rice

### SNACK

1 apple or banana

1½ tablespoons nut butter

### DINNER

1 serving **Grilled Tilapia Fillet** (page 117)

1 cup cooked green beans + 1 cup cherry tomatoes, halved

¼ cup crumbled feta cheese, sprinkled over veggies

1½ cups roasted red potatoes

### SNACK

1 cup Cheerios

8 ounces fat-free milk

# Day 54

### BREAKFAST

¾ cup old-fashioned oats cooked in 1 cup milk + water

1 apple, chopped, added to oats

1 teaspoon Splenda + 1 teaspoon cinnamon

1 tablespoon sliced almonds

(or 2 packs Quaker Weight Control Instant Oatmeal + 1 fruit choice)

### LUNCH

1 cup **Chicken Curry Salad** (page 113)

2 whole wheat pita pockets

1 cup chopped lettuce

1 cup red grapes

### SNACK

1 bag 100-calorie microwave popcorn

2 pieces low-fat string cheese

### DINNER

3 cups **Spinach Orzo** (page 135)

### SNACK

4 **Peanut Butter Balls** (page 136)

# Day 55

**1 Baked Breakfast Pepper**
(page 110)

2 slices whole wheat toast

1 tablespoon natural jam

## LUNCH

**1 Meatball Sandwich** (page 114)

1 bag Birds Eye Steamfresh Lightly Sauced
Creamed Spinach

## SNACK

¼ cup **Spicy Artichoke Dip** (page 143)

20 baby carrots

10 celery sticks

## DINNER

1½ servings **Fish and Chips Salad**
(page 122)

2 small boiled eggs, halved

## SNACK

1 cup Cheerios

8 ounces fat-free milk

# Day 56

## BREAKFAST

**1 Baked Breakfast Pepper**
(page 110)

2 slices whole wheat toast

1 tablespoon natural jam

## LUNCH

2 slices whole wheat bread

2 tablespoons peanut butter

2 teaspoons honey

1½ cups grapes

## SNACK

¼ cup **Spicy Artichoke Dip** (page 143)

20 baby carrots

10 celery sticks

## DINNER

1½ cups whole wheat spaghetti (dry noodles
with the diameter of a quarter)

¾ cup marinara sauce

3 frozen cooked meatballs

3 cups salad greens

2 tablespoons low-fat salad dressing

2 tablespoons reduced-fat Italian shredded
cheese blend

## SNACK

1 bag 100-calorie microwave popcorn

1 tablespoon mini dark chocolate chips

# Day 57

**BREAKFAST**

1 **Baked Breakfast Pepper**
(page 110)

2 slices whole wheat toast

1 tablespoon natural jam

**LUNCH**

2 cups **Black Beans and Rice**
(page 126)

**SNACK**

1 apple

2 pieces low-fat string cheese

**DINNER**

6 ounces grilled chicken breast

2½ cups **Fruit and Almond Salad**
(page 116)

**SNACK**

1 serving **Cookie Dough Yogurt**
(page 137)

# Day 58

**BREAKFAST**

1 **Baked Breakfast Pepper**
(page 110)

2 slices whole wheat toast

1 tablespoon natural jam

**LUNCH**

2 slices whole wheat bread

3 ounces reduced-sodium turkey lunch meat

2 teaspoons reduced-fat olive oil mayonnaise or spicy mustard or 1 Laughing Cow Light Cheese Wedge spread on bread

1 slice low-fat cheese

3 clementines

1 cup 100-calorie Greek yogurt

**SNACK**

30 almonds

**DINNER**

1 **Taco Salad** (page 115)

**SNACK**

1 Skinny Cow Ice Cream Sandwich

# Day 59

## BREAKFAST

1 **Breakfast Burrito** (page 109)

1½ cups melon cubes

## LUNCH

2 slices whole wheat bread

2 tablespoons nut butter

2 teaspoons honey

1½ cups grapes

## SNACK

¼ cup **Black Bean Dip** (page 143)

12 blue corn tortilla chips

2 tablespoons tomato salsa

## DINNER

4 nigiri sushi

4 spicy tuna rolls (pieces)

4 California rolls (pieces)

1 tablespoon low-sodium soy sauce

1 tablespoon wasabi

## SNACK

1 Skinny Cow Ice Cream Sandwich

# Day 60

## BREAKFAST

2 Kashi Blueberry Waffles

1 cup berries

1 tablespoon honey or pure maple syrup

1 cup cooked egg whites

1 slice low-fat cheese, in eggs

## LUNCH

2 cups **Black Beans and Rice**
(page 126)

## SNACK

1 bag 100-calorie microwave popcorn

3 clementines

## DINNER

6 ounces cooked chicken breast

1½ cups **Sweet Potato Fries**
(page 133)

1 cup steamed broccolini

1 cup mixed melon cubes

## SNACK

1 Vitalicious Vita-Top muffin or brownie

10 ounces fat-free milk

# THE GAME BUZZER

The clock has run out. The 60 days are up and the contest is over. Now what do you do?

1. Go back to the Combine section of this book located on page 43, retake your fitness test, and see how much you've improved.

2. Do your final weigh-ins.

3. Collect and tally all the data.

4. Send out any last-minute communications to let everyone know when to expect the winner to be announced.

5. Announce the winner (hopefully that's you) and distribute the trophy or prize money.

6. Set up your next competition! If you've lost all the body weight or body fat that you wanted to but you want to keep that competitive spirit alive, you can run challenges that are strictly strength and endurance based. Go back and cycle through the 60-day program, performing the Rival Strength Challenges. Compete against the others for overall best times and number of rounds performed. At the end of the 60 days, whoever had the best average scores wins.

On a personal level, you should continue to exercise and eat good, clean food.

Set another short-term goal that you can reach in 1 to 2 months. Keep in contact with your competition buddies via social media and other forms of communication to keep each other accountable. For example, weigh in every few months and set penalties (a fine, if you will) for anyone who goes over a 5-pound weight gain from the last weigh-in. Put the money into the pot as a bonus for the next competition or set a date to donate the money to a particular charity or cause.

Keep on keeping on. Live every day as if it's your last, and take care of the body that God gave you, 'cause it's the only one you've got.

# SOURCES, TEMPLATES, AND OTHER HELPFUL STUFF

**You can find a free downloadable group weight tracker and other Xcel templates from Microsoft here:**

http://office.microsoft.com/en-us/templates/group-weight-tracker-TC103987166.aspx

## Diet & Exercise Journal Template

http://office.microsoft.com/en-us/templates/results.aspx?qu=weight+loss&ex=1&av=all#ai:TC104036851|

## Food & Exercise Tracker Web Site & Apps

www.myfitnesspal.com

www.FitBit.com

www.LoseIt.com

www.LiveStrong.com

## Online Diet Tracking Web Sites

www.DietBet.com

www.stickk.com

www.skinnyo.com

hwww.healthywage.com

www.weightlosswars.com

## Fitness Stuff I Love That You May Find of Use

Cybex Arc Trainer
  www.cybexintl.com

Concept 2 Rower
  www.concept2.com

TRX
  www.trxtraining.com/

New Balance Minimus Footwear
  www.newbalance.com

PowerPlate
  www.powerplate.com/us

Muscle Milk Light
  www.musclemilk.com

Chocolate Milk
  www.GotChocolateMilk.com

Swiftwick Socks
  www.swiftwick.com

Reebok
  www.reebok.com

Buzzerk—Pre Workout Supplement
  www.completenutrition.com

Grab the Gold Nutrition Bars
  www.grabthegold.com

LifeFitness—Dual Cable Cross
  www.lifefitness.com

The Boot Campaign
  www.BootCampaign.com

Perform Better—Fitness Catalog
  www.performbetter.com

Get Uncomfortable Dare
  www.GetUncomfortableDare.com

Medals of Honor
  www.medalsofhonor.org

Reboot Combat Recover
  www.rebootrecovery.com

# FOOD DIARY

If you prefer a paper food diary to keep track of your calories, print out copies of this one.

Date: _____    **Mon  Tue  Wed  Thurs  Fri  Sat  Sun**        Weight: _____

| TIME | FOOD/BEVERAGE | AMOUNT | CALORIES |
|------|---------------|--------|----------|
|      |               |        |          |
|      |               |        |          |
|      |               |        |          |
|      |               |        |          |
|      |               |        |          |
|      |               |        |          |
|      |               |        |          |
|      |               |        |          |
|      |               |        |          |
|      |               |        |          |
|      |               |        |          |
|      |               |        |          |
|      |               |        |          |
|      |               |        |          |
|      |               |        |          |
|      |               |        |          |
|      |               |        |          |
|      |               |        |          |
|      |               |        |          |
|      |               |        |          |
|      |               |        |          |
|      |               | **Totals** |      |

**Check # 8 ounce glasses of water:** ⬭ ⬭ ⬭ ⬭ ⬭ ⬭ ⬭ ⬭ ⬭ ⬭ ⬭ ⬭

| PHYSICAL ACTIVITY | MINUTES | INTENSITY LOW/MEDIUM/HIGH | CALORIES |
|-------------------|---------|---------------------------|----------|
|                   |         |                           |          |
|                   |         |                           |          |

**How I did today:**  ☐ **Fabulous**     ☐ **Great**     ☐ **Ok**     ☐ **Will do better tomorrow**

Notes: _____

# COMPETITION BRACKETS

Here is a bracket template you can use for your competition. These types of brackets would work well if you have 8 people or 8 teams involved in the contest. Round 1 weigh-in could be at the 30-day mark. Round 2 weigh-in would be at the 50-day mark. Round 3 weigh-in at the final 60-day mark would provide a champion. If you have more teams or individuals, you would create more rounds.

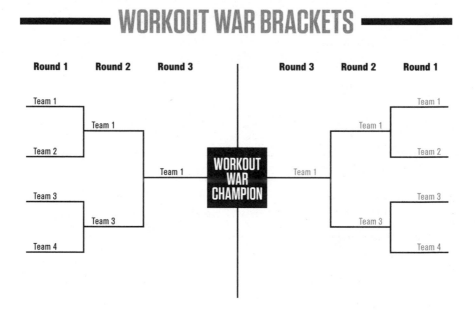

# ACKNOWLEDGMENTS

**I WOULD LIKE TO THANK GOD FOR MY AMAZING LIFE** and the many opportunities I've been given to share my love of fitness with so many incredible athletes and clients over the last twenty-plus years. With God all things are possible.

To my multitalented, multitasking wife, Amy Cotta, without whom this book wouldn't exist—it would have been nothing more than a fleeting thought. Thank you for pushing me and inspiring me to get outside of my comfort zone. Thank you for helping me to put my knowledge and sometimes-random ramblings into coherent thoughts. I love you.

I would like to thank my children: Greer, Chase, Skylar, Denver, Kali, and Tyler for their love and support. I can't imagine my life without any one of you. Everything Mom and I do, we do for you.

I would like to thank Shaquille O'Neal for writing the foreword, but more important for his friendship and being the inspiration for this book's topic.

Jeff Csatari, executive editor of Men's Health and Women's Health Books, and to the staff at *Men's Health* for being as passionate about this book as I am. Also, to my agent Linda Konner for all her hard work in bringing this project together.

I can't thank Marietta Parrish, RD, CSSD, LDN, enough for her contributions to the Lean Out Plan and recipes. And to Chef Jim O'Connell not only for kicking everyone's ass in the test group by winning it, but for his recipe contributions and input on the cooking sections.

Thank you to Alice Sullivan for her contribution to this book, and to Lululemon Athletica in Franklin, Tennessee, for providing the workout apparel used in the exercise photos.

I would also like to thank the following strength coaches, trainers, and therapists, many of whom are friends. To those I have worked with over the past 20 years, you helped to mold me into the strength coach I am today: Mark Philippi, John Binkowski, Al Caronia, Jeff Ferguson, Jerry Koloskie, Alex McKechnie, Chip Schaefer, Gary Vitti, Todd Wright, and Pete Radulavic.

Lastly, I would like to thank my parents, Marshall and Barbara Cotta, for affording me the opportunity to pursue my passion of fitness and athletics and making a career of it.

# INDEX

Boldface page references indicate illustrations or photographs. Underscored references indicate boxed text.